FOST
FOR
ADOPTION

Other books you may be interested in:

Active Social Work with Children with Disabilities
Julie Adams and Diana Leshone   9781910391945

Children Forsaken: Child Abuse from Ancient to Modern Times
Steven Walker   9781913453817

*Supporting Troubled Young People: A practical guide to
helping with mental health problems*
Steven Walker   9781912508730

Young Refugees and Asylum Seekers; The Truth about Britain
Declan Henry   9781913063979

Our titles are also available in a range of electronic formats. To order, or for details of our bulk discounts, please go to our website www.criticalpublishing.com or contact our distributor Ingram Publisher Services, telephone 01752 202301 or email NBNi.Cservs@ingramcontent.com.

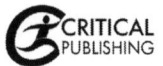

FOSTERING FOR ADOPTION

OUR STORY AND STORIES OF OTHERS

ALICE HILL

First published in 2021 by Critical Publishing Ltd

All rights reserved. No part of this publication may be reproduced, stored in a retrieval system, or transmitted in any form or by any means, electronic, mechanical, photocopying, recording or otherwise, without prior permission in writing from the publisher.

Copyright © 2021 Alice Hill

British Library Cataloguing in Publication Data
A CIP record for this book is available from the British Library

ISBN: 978-1-914171-23-9

This book is also available in the following e-book formats:
EPUB ISBN: 978-1-914171-24-6
Adobe e-book: 978-1-914171-25-3

The right of Alice Hill to be identified as the Author of this work has been asserted by her in accordance with the Copyright, Design and Patents Act 1988.

All chapter illustrations by Emma (contact details available via Critical Publishing)

Cover design by Out of House Ltd
Text design by Out of House Ltd
Project management by Newgen Publishing UK
Printed and bound in Great Britain by 4edge, Essex

Critical Publishing
3 Connaught Road
St Albans
AL3 5RX

www.criticalpublishing.com

Paper from responsible sources

For our Little J

Praise for *Fostering for Adoption*

Alice's book will be a great companion to anyone considering or starting on the Foster to Adopt process. It is well-researched and written and doesn't shy away from the many complexities and the considerations that adults must make in the best interests of children.

Sally Donovan,
Author of *No Matter What*, and Editor of *Adoption Today*

As someone who has been through a similar journey this book resonated with me. It is honest about the ups and downs and is a great, informative book for anybody thinking of taking this route or who have family or friends that are. I can say that this book will help anyone at the beginning of their journey, to help them through the process and start the lifetime of learning about how we can support our children.

Lisa Faulkner,
Author of *Meant To Be*

I thoroughly enjoyed reading this book, I found myself laughing and getting emotional throughout. As someone who has themselves been adopted, but who is also a social worker who has now adopted a child, this book is brilliant from every angle. A must read for anyone considering Fostering for Adoption.

Jo,
social worker, Midlands

This book gives a balanced and honest view of the whole Fostering for Adoption journey. It gets to the emotions and seriousness of decisions being made about children's lives. This is an important read for any potential adopter and will be on our book lists for sure.

Angi,
social worker, Adoption Tees Valley

Contents

Acknowledgements	page ix
Meet the author	page xii
Terminology	page xiii
Timeline: Alice and Will's timeline for Fostering for Adoption	page xvii
Prologue	page xviii

Chapter 1
Introduction and background to Fostering for Adoption — page 1

Chapter 2
Where our story begins:
Our decision, training and paperwork — page 18

Chapter 3
Expressing our story:
The home assessment and Adoption Panel — page 42

Chapter 4
Who will join our story?
Matching, tracking and an emotional rollercoaster — page 73

Chapter 5
The story continues:
Being matched — page 98

Chapter 6
Our story feels real:
Transition and placement — page 121

Chapter 7
Documenting the detail of our story:
The early days of Fostering for Adoption   **page 138**

Chapter 8
Retelling our story as a family of three:
Preparing for the Matching Panel   **page 157**

Chapter 9
Formalising our story:
Applying for the Adoption Order and everyday family life   **page 176**

Chapter 10
Our story can continue:
Two legally becomes three   **page 190**

Epilogue   **page 199**

References   **page 216**

Index   **page 220**

Acknowledgements

Writing the acknowledgements in a book where the author is anonymous is a little difficult. I can't name the people who have stood by us every step of the way – these people are too close to us and our story. I will, however, write this in such a way that they will know who they are.

I begin with our parents. Through the 'ups, downs ins and outs' we have laughed and cried together; we could not have done it without you. You have listened, been there for us, educated yourselves about adoption and most importantly opened your hearts to our little one.

Then to our friends. We have been overwhelmed with the support you have given us throughout this process. You have asked appropriate questions, listened, helped us make difficult decisions, given us baby clothes, cooked us meals and just been amazing. Jake is surrounded by so many people who love him and we are thankful to all of you for respecting his story and his beginning.

Next, our social workers. Two wonderful professionals taught us a lot about ourselves, asked us critical questions, listened and, above all, guided us through a complex and risky process with the upmost professionalism and care. Huge thanks to both of you. Then there is Jake's social worker, who had his best interests at heart throughout the process. You supported us on our journey to becoming parents and we will be forever thankful that you chose us as a match for him. Thank you.

I am also thankful to the other adoptees and adopters who I have met over the past few years. We have made friendships that I am sure will be lifelong. These are the people that truly 'get it' and I am sure we will turn to each other for advice in parenting our little ones. Some of these people we met through our agency and others on Instagram. In September 2020 as we reached the end of our adoption process, I was encouraged to join the Instagram community of adopters. At first, I was a little sceptical but soon came to realise that this growing community is a vital source of support and I only wish I had found it earlier. It was 'finding' this adoption community that prompted me to write this book, and indeed, where many of the case study contributors were found. Thanks to all of my followers and friends in the Instagram world – I love following your journeys and have learnt so much about adoption from this network.

Next, I would like to thank all those who have contributed case studies. Without your stories there would not be a book. I have felt passionately that this should showcase a diverse range of Fostering for Adoption stories. Over the months of writing, speaking to you, our emails and editing, I have felt an enormous sense of responsibility to your stories and the children in your care. I hope you are as proud of this book as I am. I wish all of you love and hope as you navigate your way through the system and for those of you who have been granted your Adoption Orders – wishing you love as you build your family.

I would also like to thank all the people who have been involved in the making of this book. My family, friends, social workers, adopters, adoptees, medical professionals, and academics all offered a critical eye pre-publication – with your tweaks and inputs, this book is without a doubt a stronger piece. Thank you for your insights and timely turnaround of comments.

Throughout the book there are a series of wonderful illustrations at the beginning of each chapter. Huge thanks to the artist for taking some of our very special family moments and illustrating these. All of these fit into our story so beautifully, thank you.

Next I want to thank Jake's foster carers. From the moment we met them we knew how special Jake was to them – he was their first foster child. Jane and David – Jake will grow up knowing how special you were to him, and him to you. You are the beginning of his story.

There are two people to whom Will and I are now connected via adoption – Jake's birth parents. While we have never met we hand on heart promise that Jake will grow up knowing his story and, most importantly, that he is loved.

I am now getting to the end and it is time to thank the two most important people in my life. First, Will, my husband. Will has been the rock throughout this process, the one who remained calm and offered perspective when I needed it the most. He also encouraged me to tell our story to share with you the reader. Will, you are my everything, thank you.

Then finally, our Little J. One day you will be reading the words on this page and you will come to understand why we felt we needed to share our story, our journey to finding you.

Little J, you have taught us the true meaning of love.

Meet the author

Alice Hill and her husband offer this personal account of their Fostering for Adoption experience in England. This was their route to a baby joining their family. Foster to Adopt is risky for adopters and this is their story through the journey – from the assessments, the waiting, the difficult decisions, the placement and the uncertainty. To complement their story, other families have also shared their experiences, so you as a reader get a fuller account of all it entails – the ups, the downs and everything in between.

Terminology

This book is intended for a general audience who may not be familiar with the terminology surrounding adoption. Like many people going through the adoption process, we found the terminology, language and acronyms difficult to understand at times. To help you, I have provided an explanation of all key terms that are used in the book. For other terminologies related to adoption see the Adoption Glossary provided by First4Adoption (2021).

This is a personal account of our Fostering for Adoption journey; however, I do use a range of publicly available material to ensure accuracy of the process. All references are listed at the end of the book and are available online.

Adoption Leave: adopters are entitled to the same statutory leave as birth parents (up to 52 weeks). If you are an employee, your organisation should have an Adoption Leave policy.

Adoption Order (AO): the final court order which transfers parental responsibility to the adoptive parents.

Adoption Panel: prospective adopters, through their training and assessment, work towards their Adoption Panel. This will be made up of a panel of social worker professionals and independent members, many of whom are adoptive parents. The panel will read the potential adopters' paperwork, ask a series of questions and make a recommendation to the ADM.

Agency Decision Maker (ADM): refers to a person in the adoption agency or Local Authority who has the final say on decisions which are made about prospective adopters. The ADM will take on board the recommendations from both the Adoption Panel (ADM from the agency) and Matching Panel (ADM from the Local Authority) to make a final decision on approval and matching.

Care Order (CO): a court order which takes a child into care. This gives the Local Authority shared parental responsibility for the care and welfare of the child. A Care Order ends when a child turns 18; an order is made transferring responsibility to another person (ie adopter) or the court ends the order.

Celebratory Hearing: once an Adoption Order is granted, adopters are invited to a Celebratory Hearing. This is an opportunity to meet the judge who has been involved in the case and bring the new family and social workers together to celebrate the adoption (the terminology for this varies across agencies).

Child Permanence Report (CPR): is a full report detailing the family background and the child's physical, emotional and social well-being, prepared by the lead social worker for the child. It documents from a professional perspective the decisions and reasons which have led to the child being considered for adoption.

Child Protection Register: is a list of all children and young people who have been identified as being at risk of harm.

Concurrent Planning: is a type of Early Permanence Placement. These placements have two plans for the child running *concurrently*, one to be reunified with birth family members and the other a long-term placement with the concurrent carers, via adoption.

Early Permanence Placement (EPP): is commonly used to describe Fostering for Adoption placements and Concurrent Planning Placements. Both types of placement are to ensure minimal disruption to very young children, with potential adopters accepting a child initially on a foster care basis while court proceedings decide on the outcome.

Foster care: there are many different types of foster care, including long term, short term, kinship care, emergency care, respite care, remand care, and therapeutic care.

Fostering for Adoption: is a type of Early Permanence Placement (see also Concurrent Planning). For children placed under a *Fostering for Adoption* placement the Local Authority will have determined that the child is not likely to be returned to the birth family (although there is no certainty). See Chapter 1 for a more detailed explanation of the process.

Guardian: a person whose sole responsibility is to represent the child throughout the process, put them first and think about their best interests.

Independent Reviewing Officer (IRO): the role of the IRO is to ensure the child in care is being well looked after. Their primary role is to ensure that they get to know the child or young person and, importantly, listen to their feelings throughout the process.

Interim Care Order (ICO): is a temporary court order. If social workers and the Local Authority believe a child is at risk of harm the child can be removed on an Interim Care Order.

Later Life letter: is written by the child's social worker before the case is closed. It is an in-depth account detailing the case from the perspective of the lead social worker.

Letterbox: is an agreement between the birth family and adoptive family, formally made through court, regarding the exchange of letters and communication, written within an agreed timeframe post-Adoption Order.

Life story book: an age-appropriate record to be shared by the adoptive parent(s) with the child as they grow up, so that they are aware of their background from an early age (commonly prepared by the child's social worker).

Link Maker: an online portal that enables adopters to widen their search for a child or sibling group, outside of their region.

Local Authority: has children in their care and is one type of organisation that facilitates adoption in England. Regional Adoption Agencies (RAAs) are made up of several local authorities and Voluntary Adoption Agencies (VAAs) conduct the assessments for adopters and facilitate the matching process for children in Local Authority care.

Looked After Child (LAC): refers to any child who is in the care of the Local Authority.

Looked After Child Review (LAC Review): a meeting involving all of the people who have responsibility for the welfare of the child. These meetings happen at various stages throughout the placement and the aim is to discuss the care plan and the development of the child. The meeting is chaired by the Independent Reviewing Officer (IRO) and attended by social workers, education and health care professionals, anyone with parental responsibility and, if old enough to understand, the child.

Matching Panel: is similar to the Adoption Panel, where adopters are asked questions by a panel of professionals in the social worker community – but this time in relation to a specific child or children. With Fostering for Adoption, the Matching Panel occurs after the child has been granted the Placement Order.

Mother and Baby Unit: a specialist facility for mothers who may need emotional, physical and mental support.

Pen Picture: forms part of the Prospective Adopters Report. It is a photograph and summary of the potential adopters, which the social worker then uses when they are searching for a family for the children in their care.

Placement Order (PO): is granted when the court has enough evidence to give the Local Authority permission to find an adoptive family for the child.

Prospective Adopters Report (PAR): is a document prepared by the potential adopters' social worker during the assessment phase. This document is a full account of their life (including, for example, family, health, finances, relationships, support network and employment). As part of the assessment, adopters may be asked to prepare a workbook, a series of questions that encourage self-reflection. The workbook is completed prior to Stage 2 and is used as a basis for discussion and to support the preparation of the PAR. The PAR is presented to the Adoption Panel.

Relinquished: is the term used to describe very young babies (commonly under six weeks old) where their birth parents feel that the best option for their child is adoption.

Stage 1: is the first stage of the adoption process. Prospective adopters undergo a series of checks (ie police, employment, financial, health) and a range of referees will be asked to comment on their suitability to adopt. Prospective adopters will also be expected to attend training and use this period to undertake research on adoption and all it entails.

Stage 2: is the second stage of the adoption process. Once through Stage 1, prospective adopters will be allocated a social worker who will work with them to assess their suitability to adopt.

Theraplay: is an approach to attachment building between parent and child, promoting play, trust and self-esteem.

Timeline:
Alice and Will's timeline for Fostering for Adoption

- **2018 September**
  Information evening / initial call with a social worker / Stage 1 begins

- **October**
  Stage 1 training

- **November**
  Adoption medicals / submitted Stage 1 paperwork / 'Friends and family training'

- **2019 January**
  Stage 2 begins / Stage 2 training / home assessment begins

- **May**
  Adoption Panel

- **September**
  Matched with Fostering for Adoption placement

- **October**
  Fostering for Adoption placement

- **2020 January**
  Matching Panel

- **February**
  Adoption placement

- **September**
  Adoption Order

Prologue

It is a beautiful box. Dark navy with leather handles on either side.

The week after our Adoption Order was granted we went into our local town and there it was sitting in the window of one of our favourite independent gift shops. When I saw it, I knew that this would be the box that would sit in his room and hold his story, his memories. It will tell him who he is and how he came to be with us.

We spent that afternoon filling it with his belongings – his first blanket from hospital, drawings from the foster carers' children, the cards that we were sent when he arrived, his first painting and more. As he grows, so will the special things inside.

At the moment he is too young to understand the significance of the box that sits in his room, but together we will look in it and talk about his story. I am sure that one day we will walk in to his room and he will be sitting there with it open, looking through all of his things. When this happens, we will sit by him and tell him once again how his story began, we will tell him as often as he wants to hear it, we will tell it together.

CHAPTER 1

INTRODUCTION AND BACKGROUND TO FOSTERING FOR ADOPTION

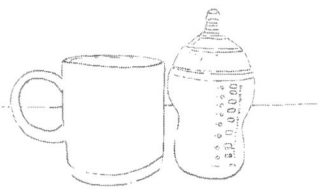

Fostering for Adoption is a route to early permanence for young children and a potential pathway to adoption – it offers stability for children at a time when they are most vulnerable. For potential adopters it is a route which they may be asked to consider by their agency during the assessment process. This book is written from my perspective as someone who, with my husband, decided this would be our route to growing our family. However, the book also includes the voices of other families who wanted to share their experiences with you. As a collective, our stories are intended to give an accessible insight into the process – the ups, downs, ins and outs of early permanence and what it can entail for potential adopters. Perhaps you have picked up this book because you are in the early days of considering adoption, or you may have already started the process and are thinking through your options, including early permanence. You may not be adopting a child yourself but you have a friend or family member who is going through the process. Or perhaps you are a social worker and are looking to understand what it feels like 'from another side'. Whatever your reason, my hope is that by the end of this book you feel that you have a more informed understanding of Fostering for Adoption – what it entails, the outcomes, and importantly, the lived experiences of adopters. Each of the families who have contributed to this book has taken a risk on behalf of a child – a child who needed love and stability in the early days and months of their life. While reading this book I want you to keep one thing in mind – the contributors agree that, despite the risk, the uncertainty and emotional toil, they would do it again; they would take the risk for the children in their care.

The process for us took two years, nearly to the day – from making an initial enquiry to our Adoption Order going through. Two weeks after we had the good news that our family of three was official we made a decision to share our story for the benefit of others. With two months of Adoption Leave remaining, while our little one slept, I started to write our story, to share with you and, one day, share with him. However, I soon decided that this couldn't just be about our story. For this to be an informative book, you need to hear about the experiences of others, not just us; every story, journey, moment, feeling and emotion will be felt differently. Every Fostering for Adoption placement is unique – there will be those cases where birth parents have expressed that they will consent to adoption, but as yet haven't officially; or where the birth parents may have already had children placed for adoption and there is strong evidence that parental circumstances have not changed; or perhaps it is the case where the risks for a newborn are too great to be placed with a birth parent or other family members and so a Fostering for Adoption placement will be made while assessments are finalised. In the majority of cases young children are placed without a Placement Order and prospective adopters take on a caring role while evidence is gathered and court proceedings take place. There are, however, a number of circumstances where young children can be placed via Fostering for Adoption with a Placement Order (as explained later on). For a detailed review of the diverse scenarios in which Fostering for Adoption placements can be made, I recommend the report by Dibben and Howorth (2017). Of course, in all of these cases

> birth parent(s) and significant wider family members [are informed] that the placement of a child on a Fostering for Adoption basis does not pre-empt the outcome of any court proceedings or, in the case of a relinquished child, alter their right to make a decision to reclaim their child at any point prior to them signing consent to placement.
> (West Berkshire Council, 2021)

This is where the risk lies – prospective adopters are taking a risk that the outcome of court proceedings may not be adoption and so the child may not remain with them.

The range of scenarios is diverse and complex, which means that we all have our own unique story to tell. There may be parts of the process that some may find relatively easy, but for others, these moments will be fraught and stressful. Given this, it is worth saying that the book may prompt tears, both happy and sad. Both individually and collectively our stories are emotional. In writing the book I have tried to strike a balance to show the everyday realities of the process. It is my hope that readers will be able to make informed choices about their own futures – using our experiences to shape your own decisions, thinking and practice.

The book is structured as a diary of our adoption process, from the day we completed our Expression of Interest, to our Adoption Order being granted – insights over a two-year period. Interspersed are case studies from others, reflecting on their own experiences and situations. This is to showcase the diversity of Fostering for Adoption. These case studies are narrated and woven into the book.

I begin with an overview of Fostering for Adoption. This material is drawn from the public domain and from insights that we received during our training. At the time of writing, there was limited information available, particularly from the perspective of adopters.

What is Fostering for Adoption?

In England, Fostering for Adoption is a route to early permanence which places young children with their potential permanent family on a foster care basis while the court decides on the plan for their future. While Fostering for Adoption is mostly considered for babies and very young children, there are cases where it is also used for older children, in the context of reducing placement moves and the individual circumstances of the child or sibling group (Dibben and Howorth, 2017). This placement option is often cited to be in the best interests of the child, so that they do not encounter multiple moves at a young age and to give stability at a time when they are most vulnerable. However, for adopters it is inherently risky; they accept a young child on a fostering basis, hoping that the outcome will be adoption.

In this situation, the rights of the young child and the birth parents take precedence, however, unlike Concurrent Planning (another type of Early Permanence Placement):

> for Fostering for Adoption placements, the Local Authority has already completed all assessments of the parents and the extended

family and has reached a clear view that the child will need to be adopted at the end of the court proceedings ... however, the judge will not have made his/her decision and sometimes there are unexpected developments such as a previously unknown relative asking to be considered.

(CoramBAAF, 2017, p 2)

Of course, making these life-changing decisions for vulnerable children *'takes time to be done in a way that is fair, lawful and evidence based'* (CoramBAAF, 2017, p 4) – which is why it is so important that early permanence is an option for these children, to reduce the risk of multiple moves and instability. In summary, Fostering for Adoption is only appropriate for those young children *'where there is clear evidence available to the Local Authority that there is very little likelihood that the birth parents can resolve their problems or that other family members can take care of the child'* (CoramBAAF, 2017, p 4). You may want to delve into case law to understand how the court considers what is in the best interest of the welfare of the child under Section 1 of the Children Act (1989) and Article 8 of the Human Rights Act (1998) – as explained by Broadhurst et al (2018, p 12), *'separation of a child from his or her parents should only be ordered by an Interim Care Order if the child's safety "demands immediate separation" or "interim protection."'* For more detail on the care proceedings surrounding newborn babies who are brought into the care system, please see Broadhurst et al (2018).

For a little more context, it is interesting to look at the history of Concurrent Planning in England. The concurrent placement of babies and young children came to the UK in 1998 (inspired by a similar route to adoption in the US) via the Goodman Project (spearheaded by the Manchester Adoption Agency). In 1999, Coram (the UK's oldest children's charity, see Coram (2021a) for more information about them and their work) began a similar initiative and they soon became known for their expertise in this field – advocating the significant benefits that this gives to babies and young children. Their work was built on the premise that *'the early environment, and the first three years of life in particular, plays a major role in shaping children's cognitive, social, economic and behavioural development'* (Laws et al, 2012, p 16). Between 2000 and 2011, Coram placed 59 children via Concurrent Planning; for a detailed analysis of the ages, profiles and permanency outcomes see the report written by Laws et al (2012).

In 2011 and 2013 there were two publications by the Department for Education which paved the way for promoting early permanence – known as Fostering for Adoption. The first report, 'An Action Plan for Adoption: Tackling Delay' (Department for Education, 2011), gave a key recommendation: to *'encourage all Local Authorities to seek to place children with their potential adopters in anticipation of the court's Placement Order'* (p 3) in recognition that this route to adoption can *'provide early stability'* (p 26) for babies and young children. The second report, 'Further Action on Adoption: Finding More Loving Homes' (Department for Education, 2013) built on this policy shift and *'set out proposals for the next steps in tackling delay so that more children can benefit more quickly from being adopted into a loving home'* (p 3).

The recommendations from these reports became cemented in law under the Children and Families Act (2014). There were two key changes to policy:

1. *Encourage Local Authorities to place children for whom they are considering adoption with their potential permanent carers more swiftly, by requiring a Local Authority looking after a child for whom they are considering adoption to place them with foster carers who are also approved prospective adopters, on a fostering basis.*

2. *Adoption leave and pay include prospective parents in the Fostering for Adoption system.*

(Children and Families Act, 2014)

It is important to note here that the legislation for Fostering for Adoption applies to England only; Wales, Scotland and Northern Ireland each have their own framework for early permanence. If you are considering early permanence as an option to adopt a child, I would recommend doing your own research on the differences in legislation across the UK. In Wales, for example, provision is termed Foster to Adopt and legally differs to Fostering for Adoption (see AFA Cymru, 2016, for a detailed explanation of the differences). The book includes a case study from Northern Ireland (early permanence via Concurrent Planning) to show how different the legislation is and why it is important that potential adopters understand these differences.

In terms of the numbers of children who are placed on a Fostering for Adoption basis, this is relatively small (compared to the number of children placed via standard adoption). Dibben and Howorth (2017) reflected on data from 2016, showing that '*320 children were placed with a foster carer who is also an approved adopter for FfA [Fostering for Adoption] or concurrent planning in the year ending March 2016*.' They also say that there are significant differences across local authorities. The latest figures (at the time of writing) showed that in 2019–20, a total of 380 children were '*in placements where the carer is also an approved adopter or where they were subject to concurrent planning*' (CoramBAAF, 2021). For a full breakdown of all government statistics related to children who are adopted and in the care system, see UK Government (2021).

One of the most frequently asked questions by prospective adopters is – '*how many of the children are returned to their birth family?*' When we were researching the process, we couldn't find this information and our agency only told us about one case (within our Local Authority), where the baby was reunified with its birth parents after six weeks. In 2017, Dibben and Howorth reported that '*there are no national figures being collected on the number of Foster for Adoption or concurrent placements where children have returned to live with birth family or where there has been a placement disruption at the request of the Foster for Adoption carer. We are not aware of any plans for this at present*' (2017, p 10). Again, at the time of writing, in 2021, I have been searching for this information, to no avail. However, a recent report by Brown and Mason (2021, p 27) reviewed the outcomes of Early Permanence Placements (EPPs) across a number of studies and found that '*the evidence-base about early permanence is weak and ... no study relating to the Fostering for Adoption model of early permanence was identified that included data on outcomes of placements*.'

In this book, I include two case studies written by families who have had the experience of a terminated placement, with the baby being returned to its birth family. From my experience of researching and talking to those who have been through the Fostering for Adoption process, these are very much in the minority. However, as you will read, many of the families in the book talk about the anxiety of not knowing if their baby is going to stay with them – this causes much uncertainty and apprehension.

The key difference between Fostering for Adoption and Concurrent Planning is that the latter has an active plan for birth family reunification (Plan A), which is being promoted alongside a Plan B, where the child would be placed for adoption. Fostering for Adoption placements are made on the basis that there is no *active* Plan A for reunification – however, this does not mean that reunification isn't possible (as explained elsewhere in this chapter). In my reading and understanding of Early Permanence Placements (EPPs), including both Fostering for Adoption and Concurrent Planning, there seems to be a blurriness around the language used. Indeed, the report by Brown and Mason (2021, p 54) concludes that because '*Concurrent Planning and Fostering for Adoption have become conflated under the umbrella term of early permanence, important distinctions between the two approaches are not always noted or understood.*'

All families in this book responded to my call for their stories on Fostering for Adoption, although some use the umbrella term Early Permanence Planning in their accounts. Each case study uses the term which is specific to their placement (ie Fostering for Adoption, Foster to Adopt, EPP, Concurrent Planning). For more information about Fostering for Adoption, please also see Coram and BAAF (2013) and CoramBAAF (2017).

In what circumstances are children placed for Fostering for Adoption?

Fostering for Adoption is intended for babies and small children where the Local Authority believes them to be at significant risk from the birth family, and care proceedings are imminent. As with some of the case studies in this book, it may be when a baby is due to be born and the professionals involved deem the risk to be too great for them to remain in the care of the birth family. In some cases, older siblings may have already been removed from the birth family into care or placed for adoption. Fostering for Adoption may enable the baby to be placed with a sibling, with the adoptive parents taking on a fostering role for the baby. Fostering for Adoption placements are also likely for relinquished babies.

What are the reported benefits of Fostering for Adoption for the child?

Fostering for Adoption, as an EPP, is intended to be in the best interest of the child. The primary aim is to ensure that young children do not endure multiple temporary foster care placements and the associated trauma that this brings. It is well documented that the first 1000 days of a child's life really matter

(RCPCH, 2018) – arguably more than any other time in life – for neurological, health and growth development. The Fostering for Adoption process ensures that delays in decision making and legal processes do not negatively impact on the child. While the social workers collate evidence and the courts consider the case, it is the potential adopters that take on a fostering role. The potential adopters are accepting the risk on behalf of the child. For the child, the outcome will be one of two – they will stay with the family who they have been placed with, which will transition from a Fostering for Adoption placement to an Adoption Placement – or they will return to their birth family.

What are the reported benefits of Fostering for Adoption for the potential adopters?

Despite the risks which adopters take when accepting a Fostering for Adoption placement there are benefits. The main benefit is having the opportunity to care for a young child, in some cases directly from hospital. For us, Fostering for Adoption gave us the potential to look after a baby, have the chance to bond and build a strong attachment – on balance, these benefits were worth the risks involved. Of course, anyone who goes into Fostering for Adoption needs to be prepared for the child to return to their birth family. I am hugely grateful to those adopters who have shared their personal experience of this – hugely traumatic for the adopters involved but, for the child, this is the best outcome – reunification with their birth family.

As you read about our story and those of others, you will get a sense of the benefits of this route to adoption, particularly the opportunities for early bonding and attachment. However, you will also read about the challenges, which are so distinct case to case. This is what prospective adopters need to think through, to decide if Fostering for Adoption is the right route for them and their family.

Is it likely that contact with birth parents will be maintained during the placement? What does this involve?

Contact with the birth family is likely to be a core feature of a Fostering for Adoption placement. Given that these children are undergoing care proceedings, it is likely that contact with birth parents will be maintained in the event of a return to the birth family. Contact with birth family ensures ongoing relationship building between birth parent and child.

The frequency of contact varies from case to case; in training we were told that this could be a minimum of once a week, to as much as seven times – depending on personal case circumstances and court orders. How contact happens also varies – some children are collected from the Fostering for Adoption carers and escorted to a contact centre, and others are taken directly to the contact centre by their carers. The timing of contact also varies as does the location; for some it could mean an hour's drive to a contact centre, a two-hour visit and an hour to return home. The logistics and emotional toil of this should not be underestimated. This is a huge commitment – particularly in the early days of caring for a baby or young child. Fostering for Adoption carers have no say in the frequency, timing or logistics of contact; this is directed by the court and is non-negotiable. Most Fostering for Adoption children will also have a final contact session with birth parents and, not withstanding risks and confidentiality, there would be an opportunity for birth parents and adoptive parents to meet, once the placement changes from a Fostering for Adoption placement to an Adoption Placement.

While contact with birth parents can be exhausting and emotional, families in this book have also reflected on this positively. The face-to-face contact with birth parents can bring life story work alive – they can get to know the birth parents' mannerisms and stories about them; this will be vital in future conversations with their little ones. For birth parents too, this is important – as for them, they may gain reassurance that their baby is loved and cared for by the potential adopters. In this book there are numerous accounts of contact; how it is managed and experienced varies substantially and I hope you get a good sense of what this could involve from reading these stories.

How much information do Fostering for Adoption carers receive about the child?

With Fostering for Adoption placements there is often limited information available to the prospective carers primarily due to impending court orders and confidentiality. All information given prior to placement may be verbal, rather than seeing the full reports and histories of the child and the families. As recognised by Families for Children (2021), *'there is a slight risk that at the point of Placement Order, when full detailed information becomes available, that Fostering for Adoption carers may feel they cannot proceed to adoption.'* You will get a good sense of the information that we were presented with during the matching stage of our journey. A life-changing decision was being made on verbal and sometimes limited information – this was stressful and emotional.

There may be scant information available for babies that are placed via Fostering for Adoption. Of course, the health of the child may not be known for days, weeks, months or even years after being placed. The impact of domestic violence (see the case on page 34), drugs, alcohol abuse in utero and genetic conditions may not be evident at birth – these are further risks to be considered.

We have heard that the Fostering for Adoption process is emotional, why is this?

I have hinted already that this process is emotional. As you read our story, and those of others, you will see how the uncertainty and risks associated can take their toll. When we made the decision to be considered for Fostering for Adoption, we read this quote from another adopter *'it is not for the fainthearted or overly emotional'* (CoramBAAF, 2017, p 5). I would put myself in the 'emotional' category; however, my husband, Will, the calm one, is a good counterbalance. Emotional triggers come from the uncertainty of the process, the not knowing if this small child in your care is going to be forever, uncertainties surrounding the lack of information shared on placement and contact with birth family, which can be exhausting and draining. Of course, these are only a few aspects – the everyday ins and outs of the process, the paperwork, the meetings and the pure love you have for this child is emotional.

What are the main responsibilities of a Fostering for Adoption carer?

The babies and young children on Fostering for Adoption placements are *'some of the most vulnerable in the care system'* (Coram, 2021b), so their care needs to be prioritised by those looking after them.

When a Fostering for Adoption placement is accepted, one person becomes the foster carer and is legally required to undertake various caring responsibilities associated with the placement. In our case, we decided that since I would take a year of Adoption Leave and for the Fostering for Adoption period, I would be the primary carer. The named carer has to attend all necessary appointments in relation to the welfare of the child and is expected to document, in detail, their daily activities and milestone progress.

As I have explained, for Early Permanence Plans, including Fostering for Adoption, there may be an expectation of contact between the young child and their birth family (with the rationale that if the young child were to be reunified with their birth family, then there would be some continuity of care). The Fostering for Adoption carer has a legal duty to support this process and attend the sessions (see Brown and Mason, 2021, for further insight into contact arrangements).

We are thinking about Fostering for Adoption, what are the potential considerations when looking at profiles?

There is nothing that prepares you fully for when you 'get the call' about a Fostering for Adoption placement. Notebook at the ready, you write down all the key details and then you are given a limited window to confirm your intention – go ahead and meet the social worker or say no to the placement. During our training we were given a list of questions to have to hand when you are in this moment:

- What historical evidence is held on file by social services, have other children previously been removed and what was the outcome?
- What were the outcomes of any previous parenting assessments?
- Have assessments been done or are they being done on the extended family? What are the timelines for these assessments?
- If the birth mother was known to misuse substances during pregnancy, what medical assessments have been done and what is the medical prognosis?
- What current and future needs is the child likely to have?
- How confident are the professionals on the likely outcome of the Fostering for Adoption placement?

- What are the views of the independent reviewing officer, the legal team, the guardian?
- What are the plans for contact with birth family?

(Notes taken from agency training)

As you read our story and hear about the Fostering for Adoption placements we were offered, you will get a sense of the complexity of the cases, and the speed at which decisions have to be made.

What is the process leading up to a Fostering for Adoption placement?

For those young children who have been identified as being at risk of harm, a series of assessments will determine if Fostering for Adoption may be a suitable pathway for the child. Often these assessments happen pre-birth with family members. If these are negative, in that there are significant concerns for the welfare of the child, then the social worker team will put in place a plan. In discussion with the legal team, a decision is made to determine if the threshold is met to start care proceedings. Depending on the outcome, birth parents would be informed of the process and the intention for Fostering for Adoption.

Young children that are relinquished can also be placed for Fostering for Adoption. In these cases there is often a lower risk of harm from the birth parents. If a decision is made to relinquish before birth, they will be asked to take part in counselling to ensure they are making the right decision for them and their baby. If, after the birth, they still want to pursue then they are given the option of either the baby entering mainstream fostering or being placed on a Fostering for Adoption basis. In these cases where birth parents have parental responsibility, consent for adoption cannot be made until six weeks post-birth – so in effect, birth parents have this time to change their mind. In these cases, even when consent has been given, birth parents can change their mind right up until the Adoption Order.

Our story

I hope that now you have some sense of what Fostering for Adoption can involve. It is time for me to share our story and our journey through the process. Before I start, a little context is needed. Will and I sat in a restaurant in

Italy and after four years of marriage and thirteen years together we decided that now was the time to start to try for a family. This was a big moment. We were both in jobs, in careers which were progressing in ways in which we enjoyed and were excited by. I felt I was at a good stage: I was nearing the end of a project, and the timings would 'work' – fitting in my job with a planned pregnancy.

This is not a book about infertility, so it is not the place to go into the details of the four years we had of trying to conceive. We will leave it that we tried, but we ended this phase with the sadness of multiple miscarriages and depressed by the success rates of in vitro fertilisation (IVF). We had always talked openly about adoption and in the summer of 2018, on holiday in Norfolk, we made the decision – to draw a line under fertility treatment and to make enquiries about adoption. We begin our story in Chapter 2, the day we attended an open evening at our Local Authority to talk through the options of growing our family through adoption. We actively made a decision to begin this book at this stage of our journey. We recognise that each person considering Fostering for Adoption will have their own story and reasons for wanting to understand more about this pathway to adoption. Whatever your background and personal circumstances, we hope that you will be able to relate to the issues raised in this book – both ours as a couple and those of the other families who have contributed.

This is our story, mainly written through my eyes. While Will and I went through all of this as a couple, I am the one who loves to journal and write down every detail. The book has however been edited by both of us to ensure it is an accurate representation of both of our experiences. I write it as a diary, documenting our account of the process of Fostering for Adoption. This is as close to reality as I can share with you; all dates and names have been changed to ensure the anonymity of our family, friends, Local Authority, social workers, foster carers, health visitors, birth family and of course our Little J. Of course, you will hear more about Jake as the book progresses but for a little insight, Jake came into our care at six months old, a beautiful, happy and content baby. He is now two and is the centre of our world. This book is primarily about the journey through the adoption process, so while of course we talk about Jake, we have not shared his full story. Outside of social services and us as a couple, nobody knows his full story – and it is not our story to share. This is his beginning and as he grows up he will be the keeper of his story and share it as he feels comfortable doing so. In the chapters which document the days and months between his arrival and our Adoption Order, we have also not written about every meeting with social workers and adoption professionals, in an attempt not to write repetitive accounts.

We have tried to be as open and honest as possible. Fostering for Adoption is still in its infancy and the willingness to place children on a Fostering for Adoption placement varies across local authorities and adoption agencies. When we were doing our own research, this is the book we wanted to read; a book with real-life accounts of the process to be able to make an informed decision on the path to adoption we were thinking of taking. Through our account we hope you get a sense of the everyday realities of Fostering for Adoption, a process intended to be in the best interests of the child, one which is risky, beautiful, amazing and fraught rolled into one.

You also need to bear in mind that this is an account of *our* process. While there are legal and practical consistencies across agencies, this is our pathway, our training and our outcome. You will be able to get a good sense of our journey and you may be able to see parallels in your process (if you have already started).

You will get a good sense of who we are as a couple, what worries us, what excites us and more. To set the scene I share below an excerpt from one of the initial documents we were asked to prepare for our social worker. Here we reflect on us as a couple, how we are similar, how are different and how we work together:

> *Will and I are similar in many ways, we are both adventurous, happy in our professional careers, have a love of travel and exploration. We are both ambitious and encourage each other to achieve our personal and collective goals. We are both committed to our families and appreciate all that our families do for us. In terms of differences, I am more of a worrier and Will always has perspective. If I am ever worried about something I run it past him; 9 times out of 10 he will say, it's fine and I don't need to worry about it. If Will tells me to worry, then I should worry. I would say that I am more of a planner and Will has more spontaneity – this is also a good mix. We are a team – working our way through life and all that it throws at us.*

As I read this statement written in the early stages of our adoption training and assessment, I realise how important these qualities have been as we have moved through the process – through the anxiety, the emotion, the pure joy of the journey we have been on.

I write our story chronologically, how Fostering for Adoption happened for us, from the outset of the adoption process to the decision making, Fostering for Adoption placement, Adoption Placement and finally the Adoption Order. The notes that I wrote at the time formed the basis of the script for this book. So too have a series of voice diaries that I made during the matching phase of the process – the raw emotion seeps out of the pages – mainly because it is written directly from my feelings at the time.

Of course, our story is only one account of Fostering for Adoption. When we decided to share our story we were clear that this book couldn't just be about our experience. If you are picking this book up to learn more about Fostering for Adoption, you need to hear about more than one family. In writing this book I was overwhelmed by the support from others – they wanted to share part of their story too. We felt it was important to include a range of experiences, from those right at the start of their journey, to those undergoing the assessment process, the matching, placement and post-Adoption Order. These stories are interspersed throughout the book, showcasing their diverse experiences of early permanence – from experiences of sibling placements, newborn babies, twins, drug withdrawal, managing risks, contact with birth family, relinquished children, terminated placements and life story work. Next I introduce these families to you, a diverse group of adopters representing different backgrounds and demographics, and their contribution and chapter(s) in which they appear. All families have contributed using pseudonyms.

- **Hannah and Claire** are second-time adopters. They adopted a little girl three years ago. She arrived to them on a Foster to Adopt placement as a one-week-old baby. In their case study, they reflect on the risks they experienced throughout the process (Chapter 5) and caring for a baby withdrawing from drugs (Chapter 4).

- **Elaine and James** are based in Northern Ireland and are also repeat adopters, with the same birth mother. Both babies were placed on Concurrent Planning placements, one at seven weeks old and the other at seven days. They reflect on their experience of repeat adopting (Chapter 10); contact, visits and paperwork (Chapter 7); and risk during the process (Chapter 4).

- **Charlotte and Richard** draw on their experience of Foster to Adopt with siblings. Their boys were placed weeks apart, one from foster care (aged one) and a newborn from hospital. They have written case studies on caring for a baby a few days after birth (Chapter 3), contact with birth parents (Chapter 7), contact with older siblings (Chapter 9), a sibling placement (Chapter 8), responsibilities as foster carers (Chapter 7) and uncertainty (Chapter 8).
- **Sarah and Alex** are currently in the matching phase, waiting for a placement. They have had the unfortunate experience of a terminated Foster to Adopt placement with a relinquished baby (Chapter 5). They also reflect on what is needed to be prepared (Chapter 4) and the emotional struggles of quick decisions and false hopes (Chapter 4).
- **Nellie and Louis** waited for over a year for their EPP, so speak about the uncertainty they experienced during this phase (Chapter 4). They were placed with a three-month-old girl and they reflect on the positive experience they have had in maintaining contact with birth siblings (Chapter 9).
- **Rachel** accepted a six-week-old boy on a Foster to Adopt placement. She writes about how she dealt with work in preparing for an imminent arrival (Chapters 4 and 5), the first two weeks (Chapter 7), the logistics involved with contact (Chapter 3) and the life story book (Chapter 3).
- **Beatrix and Thomas** had a whirlwind of an experience (Chapter 3), being matched straight after their Adoption Panel. They accepted a sibling Foster to Adopt placement with a five-day-old and 22-month-old. They reflect on the uncertainties surrounding their placement (Chapters 7 and 10) and their experiences of contact with birth parents (Chapter 7).
- **Katie and Jack** share their experience of the early days of their Foster to Adopt placement, bringing a two-day-old boy home from hospital (Chapter 4).
- **Joanne and John** were also placed with a newborn baby, a one-day-old boy on a Concurrent/Fostering for Adoption placement (Chapter 4). Their baby was relinquished at birth and they speak about not having contact with his birth mother (Chapter 3).
- **Paul and John** accepted a two-week-old baby from hospital on an EPP only to find out that a re-assessment of a family member would lead to the baby being returned to the birth family, three months after placement (Chapter 5).

- **Sam and Alexander** initially didn't want to do Foster to Adopt; for them it was too risky. However, they found themselves accepting a six-month-old baby girl, with the reassurance that all would be fine. However, with various delays and parental re-assessments, they speak about falling into a Foster to Adopt placement and the risky situation they find themselves in (Chapter 8).
- **Jessica and Mark** accepted twin boys at 12 days old. They speak about making the decision (Chapter 2) with their birth children (Chapter 3), the early days of their EPP (Chapter 3) and contact and life story work (Chapter 9).
- **Kristie** also accepted twins aged six weeks on an EPP. She reflects on being a single adopter and the importance of her support network (Chapter 2) and getting ready for their arrival (Chapter 5).
- **Nicole and Paulo** are in Stage 2 of the process and are weighing up if Fostering for Adoption is suitable for them to grow their family. After years and years of heartache in trying to conceive, they are not sure if they are resilient enough to cope with the uncertainty of the process (Chapter 3).
- **Louise and Ian** were placed with a three-month-old baby girl on a Foster to Adopt placement. They reflect on the contact process while the parental assessments were being carried out and the practicalities of these sessions (Chapters 3 and 7).
- **Louise and Nick** share their experience of accepting a two-day-old, relinquished baby. They expected this to be a straightforward Foster to Adopt placement but they document the rollercoaster of uncertainty that they experienced (Chapter 5).

As you read our story and those of others you will see that you have to go into this believing that you and the child(ren) in your care are in this together. You have to hold on tight, ride the waves of uncertainty and hope that your life together can continue. Yes, it is risky, yes, it is uncertain, but all being well it will be the start of something beautiful.

CHAPTER 2

WHERE OUR STORY BEGINS: OUR DECISION, TRAINING AND PAPERWORK

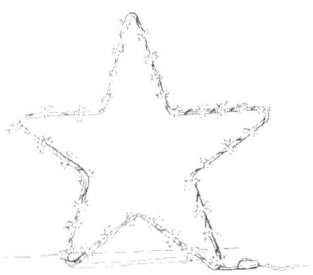

This is the start of our story. It was summer and we were on holiday in Norfolk – we had time to sit, think, chat and reflect. Over the past few months, I had tentatively, with intrigue, been scrolling through our Local Authority website pages on adoption. As for many, holidays are often the time when big decisions are made. It was mid-holiday, a Thursday morning, the sun was shining – we sat in one of our favourite cafés, ordered a pot of tea and a slice of cake, then we did it. We peered at my phone and completed the online 'Expression of Interest' form to our Local Authority – and just like that, with a click of a button, the process had begun. We held hands and smiled; this was it, we were on the way to growing our family. We begin this chapter from the day of our first information evening. That morning I wrote a note and left it on the kitchen table; it said 'I love you. This is the start of a wonderful, beautiful but equally terrifying journey ... see you there.'

2018

4 September

It is 4:06pm – in an hour and a half we will be sitting in our first adoption meeting. I am excited, nervous and terrified, all wrapped in to one. A conveyor belt of questions is running through my head: Will they like us? What are they looking for? What are they going to ask us? When will we be able to start? What will the other families be like? Over the past week I have felt pure excitement that this is the start of something new, the start of a process which will more than likely end with a positive outcome. We have had daily conversations about the everyday acts of parenthood that we are most looking forward to – working on a jigsaw, doing homework, sitting at the kitchen counter, going to the park, holidays with family and of course cuddles. For years now, we have enviously watched our friends, family, neighbours and strangers become parents – now it might be our time; this is exciting, yet hugely daunting.

Yesterday I was at a work event to give a presentation; as I drove to the venue, I cried. An overwhelming feeling took me off guard. The last time I was there, I started to miscarry. I had to put on a brave face and just do it, knowing that we were losing our baby. I had parked this experience in the back of my mind, but yesterday, driving back to the place, brought it back. The tears rolled down my cheeks as I thought about what we had been through and what we were about to embark on.

Who knows what is going to happen tonight, but for now I hope that Will and I can be ourselves and come out of the meeting with more information about the process and, above all, be excited about our future family. We feel prepared for this initial meeting but realise this is only the tip of the iceberg – we have so much to learn on our journey to parenthood.

Somewhere out there, there may be one or two children that will become part of our family – this feels overwhelming – just breathe and smile.

5 September

Will and I met at the council office, waited in the Reception and were soon shown to a meeting room. There were eight other potential adopters, everyone seated in a semi-circle. It was hard not to wonder about the circumstances of the others in the room. Before the meeting started we were able to chat to those sitting next to us, and we introduced ourselves. It soon became apparent that people come to adoption for diverse reasons. One couple was perhaps in their late forties, they already had a 16-year-old daughter; another had been through five unsuccessful rounds of IVF; and there was a single man who had brought a friend along for support. The meeting was run by the manager and a social worker in the adoption team, the purpose was purely information sharing – we all sat and took it in. Of course, I had come prepared with a brand new 'Adoption notebook'. After a few minutes I couldn't help but notice that no one was taking any notes. I felt self-conscious reaching for my notebook and pen but the inner notetaker in me couldn't attend this meeting and not write anything. The main messages were as follows:

About potential adopters: There was lots of information about different types of adopters. They offered reassurance that there is not a stereotypical adopter family. I felt this was positive. There was, however, a strong emphasis on childcare experience, the point being made that if you don't have any, then you need to make arrangements to be able to demonstrate that you have had responsibility for children in your care, in some capacity. We were also advised to do as much research and reading as possible at this stage on all aspects of the process, including attachment, drug withdrawal, contact and life story work – we were told that later on in the process our assessing social worker would need to see evidence of our knowledge base around these issues. In terms of practicalities of employment and Adoption Leave, there was a strong emphasis on adopters (one adopter if in a couple) needing to take 12 months of leave, post-placement. This is a requirement from our agency, to allow for the process to be hopefully complete (in terms of the Adoption Order) and to give maximum time for bonding and attachment.

About the process: There are two key phases which happen before you can become approved adopters, which are known as Stage 1 and Stage 2. Stage 1 includes an initial home visit which opens the door to a large amount of paperwork, finance details, DBS checks, medicals and six references, two from family and four from friends. In Stage 2 potential adopters are allocated a social worker and then a series of home visits and assessments take place. The meetings are designed to cover a range of topics for the social worker to get to know you and assess your suitability as a potential placement. These are in-depth and personal for the social worker to be able to write a Prospective Adopters Report (PAR), a detailed account to present to the panel. There wasn't much information about what happens after the panel, although this would be many months away, so one step at a time. We were also informed about Fostering for Adoption, a specific pathway. We went into this meeting thinking that 'babies were not an option'; we imagined and expected to be placed with a toddler. However, our adoption agency seemed to be pushing this newer route to adoption, one which is in the best interests of the child. They asked us to keep our minds open to this route to adoption and do our research on the risks and uncertainty that it can involve. As soon as I heard about it, I was excited. I looked over to Will, I wasn't sure what he would think of it – but both of us smiled, you know that *'let's do it'* kind of smile – perhaps we could do this.

About post-adoption support: At the end of the meeting the focus shifted to post-adoption support. Of course this is tied to government funding and priorities, so is likely to look quite different when we may need support down the line. We were also told that social workers stay with adoptive families for 12 months after the Adoption Order goes through, to ensure families are getting the support they need.

The hour and a half session was informative and very well done. There were however two points that worried me. As the presentation came to a close I turned to Will and we shared our concerns. We decided it was best to speak with one of the social workers to check we would be able to progress. As the group filtered out of the room, we stayed behind to ask our questions. Our first concern related to the timings of previous fertility treatment. The agency rule was that you have to be six months post-fertility treatment before embarking on Stage 1 of the process – this is to be sure that adoption is the right journey for you, and emotionally, you are in a strong place. In the presentation, emphasis was put on the grieving process you go through when you can't naturally conceive or keep a baby to full term. We understand this and have been there, indeed, will always be there in some way. We have read books on grieving the loss of a baby and I have had a necklace made in memory of our little ones – our experiences of baby loss have shaped who we are today. They will always be part of us. We asked for clarification on the timeline of being post-fertility treatment. The social worker told us that we have to be clear of intracervical insemination (ICI) and IVF and not under the care of a consultant. This is the bit I am worrying about; while we are six months clear of treatment, technically we are still under the care of a consultant. To be able to progress I need to write to the consultant and this needs to happen before we have our adoption medical as it is at this stage that our GP will need to declare if we are undergoing any fertility treatment. This scares me – even though we are 100 per cent committed, now we have made the decision to adopt, withdrawing from consultant care seems so final and very much the end of that stage of our journey.

The other concern that we have is our planned kitchen extension, the last room in our house to be renovated. During the presentation, the manager said *'potential adopters can't be undergoing any major home renovations.'* This is when the panic set in; how major is major? Potential adopters have to have a health and safety home inspection during Stage 2 and any house renovations need to be completed before you begin the process. We discussed our plans and timings with the social worker; she didn't seem to think there would be a problem, as long as the work would be done by Easter next year. There was, however, a clause: it will be our allocated social worker that will have the final say. We will have to keep our fingers crossed that they will be sympathetic to this and will be able to see from the rest of the house that we will get the job done.

Once we were home we made dinner and talked through our impressions, concerns, anxieties and excitement. Our overriding feeling was excitement – this is it, this is the start. We talked about Fostering for Adoption; we are interested, despite the risks it may entail. We have decided to keep our options open at this stage.

In terms of next steps, we have been told that within five days we will receive a call from a social worker to have an initial discussion about our intention to adopt. We gave them my number, as I am more likely to be able to answer a call while at work. This means the pressure is on. It is my responsibility to get us past the first hurdle, this relies on me – it is an important phone conversation.

I have been buzzing since last night. This feeling is equivalent to when I found out I was pregnant last year, pure excitement and joy of what was to come. In some way, this is how I know that this is the right thing for us to do. After work I started to tidy the spare room in preparation for the home visit, premature I know – given that we haven't even had the initial call. Will had a tough day at work so I had to temper my excitement when he got home. Unfortunately, the social worker didn't call today, hopefully the phone will ring tomorrow.

6 September

Today I am spending the day in one of my favourite cafés. I am incredibly lucky that I can be flexible with my working locations. I arrive at 9am, take up my usual spot and work through to 4pm, almost unaware of the comings and goings of parents, grandparents, toddlers, babies, work meetings and friends who meet for breakfast, brunch, lunch and afternoon tea. Beside me is my phone – I stare at it, willing it to ring.

During my lunch break I thought it would be worth making some notes to refer to when the social worker calls. I made a list of all of our childcare experiences; it is quite extensive, surely we have enough? Just after lunch, it rang. I calmly answered. It was intense, a 50-minute call, all about us. The lady was lovely, relaxed in her questioning and in the background I could hear her typing away. In the back of my mind I was hoping I was saying the 'right things'. She began by giving more information about the process; cue more notes being written in my notebook. She asked about our relationship as a couple, our journey to deciding to adopt. She didn't ask specifically about being under the care of a fertility consultant at this stage, but ringing the clinic was on my to-do list. She asked if we had done any research and asked which books we had read, I mentioned *No Matter What* by Sally Donovan (2013); tap, tap, tap, she made a note of this. She also asked if either of us had lived in any other countries. I mentioned that I had done short stints living in the USA, India and Vanuatu. She said that during the assessment process we might need police checks from each of these countries. My heart sank, particularly regarding Vanuatu and India – I know what the everyday bureaucracy is like in these countries, this is something that could take months and months to sort out.

It took me off guard when she asked me what age of child we would be interested in adopting. I wasn't really expecting to be asked this so early on in the process. I said we were keen on Fostering for Adoption and she wanted to know if we were aware of the risks and asked what drew us to it. I was honest – we were drawn to the possibility of caring for a young baby and we also liked the child-centric ethos behind the process. The conversation then progressed to our careers and the work we have done over the years with children. I explained that we both have experience of working with children who have experienced neglect and abuse and it is these life experiences that have played a part in our decision to adopt. In talking about my work and the amount of travel I have done in recent years, I emphasised that I wouldn't be doing any long-term, extensive travel once we are placed with a young child – clearly our personal and professional priorities will shift when children are in our lives.

At the end of the call she asked if we had any questions or anything we felt she needed to know. I crossed my fingers and mentioned the kitchen and our plans for the renovation in the New Year. She was reassuring although she added in the same caveat – that it would be the decision of our assessing social worker; if they feel that the work may not be completed before the panel, then we would have to press the pause button on the process. I made a mental note to make an urgent call to our builder.

In preparation for the social worker call Will and I had written a list of questions to ask, mainly relating to the ins and outs of the Fostering for Adoption process. However, as the conversation progressed I decided that this call wasn't the place to ask these questions. I am sure we will have ample opportunity when we attend the training sessions.

I was exhausted but beaming – we had got over the first hurdle. She confirmed that we are able to progress to a home visit, arranged for 18 September. There was, however, one thing that worried me – during the call, despite our experience of working with and looking after children, she emphasised that we haven't had a child to stay overnight in our house, on their own. Yes, we have our friends' children to stay, but always with their parents. I have to say though, as youth leaders, where we have looked after 20-plus children, for a week, overnight, and are completely responsible for them – surely this 'counts'?

I made two calls before I left the café. First to Will. I knew he wouldn't be able to answer the call, so I left a message to let him know how it went. The second, to our builder. I needed to emphasise the importance of our timeline, and why we don't have room for delay. He was delighted for us and told us that he and his wife are currently going through the assessment process to be foster carers, what a reassuring coincidence. He guaranteed us that everything would be completed by Easter next year, in time for our home assessment and our all-important Adoption Panel. Fingers crossed that everything goes to plan.

7 September

This morning I rang our fertility clinic. This feels such a massive step. That is it, a one-minute call draws a line through this phase of our life – we are no longer under the care of a fertility consultant.

14 September

It is over a week since I have written an entry. We have had a busy week getting ready for our home visit. The day after the social worker called we wrote a list of all the house jobs that we have been meaning to do for the past few months. Now we have purpose, a drive to get them done and tick them off the list. We put pictures up on the walls and finished several painting jobs. It felt good to be getting ready. I have also cleaned out the fridge and the cutlery drawer. My irrational self says the social worker may take a peak in the fridge or the cupboards – whereas my rational self tells me off for being ridiculous – but as I keep saying to Will, you never know, and it does need to be done.

This week we also made the decision to tell a few more people, a few colleagues and close friends. Their reactions have been nothing but supportive – we are so lucky to be surrounded by such lovely, understanding people. Four days until our home visit, we are so excited, but trying to keep our cool.

15 September

It is 4:17am and I am wide awake. I have been tossing and turning for hours, so have decided to get up. I finished the ironing, went through some work emails and have now made myself a cup of tea. I can't decide if I am nervous or excited. I keep going over the questions we may get asked, playing out our responses. I am trying to imagine what the social worker will look like, will they like us, where will they sit and the all-important question, should we offer cake? (The amount of time we deliberated this was really quite ridiculous!) Last night we went out for dinner with Will's parents. We chatted lots about the future and them being on hand for nanny and grandad duties – I can't wait for our parents to be grandparents to a future little one. We also made a decision – a cake will be made!

16 September

Today we had arranged to meet some friends of friends in a local park. Two years ago they adopted a beautiful little girl. It was amazing, we went for a long walk and chatted about all aspects of the adoption process. We feel like we have had a peak into what our life could be like and we are buzzing.

17 September

Tomorrow is our first home visit. We have cleaned, hoovered and tidied, all forms are filled in and the cake is in the oven. I am so excited but also nervous, fingers crossed it all goes well.

18 September

I was nervous waiting for the social worker to arrive, Will, of course, was calm and collected. Thank goodness one of us was. She arrived promptly at 2pm, we welcomed her in and offered her a drink which meant we were able to chat before starting the meeting (for those interested, in all our nervousness we forgot to offer the cake!). We soon found out she was a youth leader, so we had an instant connection. We were soon talking about all things youth volunteering related. Once we were sitting in the living room, she launched in with the big question, 'why adoption and why now?' After our answer about growing our family and it being the right time to start the process, we moved on to other questions about our careers and experiences of working with young people. She was very keen to know about our support network and how they would be there to help us at various stages of the journey, from the emotional to the practical. After about two hours of going through the details, dispelling our myths and talking about options, she said we needed to talk about 'next steps' – I gave Will a prod, as if to say, well that sounds like a good sign. She explained that next we needed to organise our medicals and contact our referees to ask if they would be willing to support our application to adopt. Before she left she asked to have a look around the house. As we walked from room to room I thought to myself that those hours that we spent cleaning were well spent.

We were buzzing, it went so well. Just before she left, she informally told us that she is recommending that we go through to the next stage of the process, and we should get written confirmation in the next few days. While she was with us she even rang the office to see if we could get onto the October training course; we took that as another good sign. Bubbling with excitement, we went to see our next-door neighbour to ask if she would be one of our references, and she kindly agreed. We feel like we are a few steps closer. A celebratory dinner was in order; in less than a year we could have a baby living with us.

27 September

The past week has been busy, so I haven't had much time for any journaling – I have had time to think though. I am making sure I try to go for a run several times a week. I find this time really great for some headspace – thinking through the process, the complexities and a mental 'to-do' list.

On Sunday I met some friends for brunch. As I walked to meet them I glanced into a department store window display. I smiled. I was looking at a beautiful, grey, wooden cot. Just a few months ago, this sight would have hit me in the pit of my stomach. I would have been sad. Now, as I walked on my own past the store a smile crept across my face. I knew our turn was on the horizon. On Monday we officially had the news that we were through to Stage 1; this means that we can now officially register our interest to adopt. The paperwork now begins; on Tuesday evening it took us in excess of five hours to pull together all the information needed, from previous addresses to medical information, relationships and travel histories. We submitted all the information on Wednesday morning and were told that we will receive our pack about the training course within five days. The course we are booked onto is over an hour and a half journey from our home. It is for three full days and we have decided to book a hotel and stay the night. This will give us time and space for a proper debrief session and dinner after each day. We are really looking forward to it, particularly meeting new people who are at the same stage as us, learning more about the process and hearing from other adopters about their experiences.

We decided that we also needed to have a meeting with our respective bosses at work to talk through our plans for the adoption and parental leave. I was so nervous about my meeting but I need not have been, it went really well and I felt that my workplace will support me through the process. They also agreed to be one of my referees (a requirement of the referee process). We spent time looking at our workplace and statutory Adoption Leave, any allowances for training and matching, and specific requirements of the Fostering for Adoption process.

30 September

Last night one of our family friends came to visit with her daughter. We had a wonderful evening catching up and had dinner together at our local pub. They were delighted to hear about our intention to adopt.

Over the past few weeks, we have been doing lots of adoption research, in preparation for our training and individual assessments – focusing on attachment and trauma in childhood. From what we have learnt so far, there are a few important messages and three points have stuck with us. The first is that adopters, as parents, should not deny their child the trauma of loss – a child of any age who has been through the care system will, to varying degrees, and in different stages of their life, experience trauma. It is the responsibility of the parents to support the child through this as they learn about themselves and their story. Second, despite birth parents often not having the emotional, physical, financial and psychological tools to care for their baby, they love their children. Third, leading up to a child being adopted, some for many months, if not years, will have been surrounded by a huge web of people including birth parents, siblings, extended family, foster carers, social workers, health visitors, educational psychologists and more. When a child is placed with their adoptive parents, many of these connections are severed and the child will experience loss on many levels. There is much more for us to learn about attachment building, to understand the different forms and experiences of attachment and how to build attachment in the days, months and years after placement.

2 October

We have started to fill in our workbooks – this document will be used to inform our Prospective Adopters Report (PAR). The workbook is a 30-page document containing 50 questions, all about us as a potential adopter; we have to complete one of these each. This is intended as a *'tool for you to begin to consider your own strengths, capacities and identification of issues to be explored in your home study assessment ... it asks you to think about the changes that adopting a child will bring and any adjustments that will be needed in your lifestyle'* (Agency paperwork).

We are working on our reports independently; once we have a first draft we will compare notes and read each other's. It is quite hard to know what to write and how much. I don't want to go overboard, but also I don't want the social workers to think we haven't worked hard on this. I am trying to answer a few questions each evening. I look ahead to what questions are next and can then spend the day mulling them over. I was working at home today, so when I had finished I sat by the fire and began to write. An hour later Will arrived home from work – he found me in a flood of tears, I was so upset. Some of the questions really prompt you to think differently about your own childhood and adult life. Doing the workbooks is emotional and draining. I can only really work on it for a couple of hours at a time. I thought it would be interesting to share a couple of the questions and how I have responded, for anyone else facing the task of completing their PAR. Below is an example, related to parenting styles and childhood experiences:

What elements of having been parented/cared for would you like to repeat as a parent?

Unfaltering love: whatever happens when you are a child, you should be loved. Children make mistakes, we all do – having love as a solid grounding is important.

Support: growing up can be difficult, it has challenges. My parents were always there for me to show me the way and give options for how to navigate situations.

Routine: we always had a routine in our household, this has shaped how I am today. I see routine as being important for structure and self-worth.

How do you think your childhood experiences have shaped you as an adult?

I think there are so many fragments of childhood that make their way into our adult lives. Most importantly, in relation to our intention to adopt, is my experience of being raised by my step-father. Some years after the death of my birth father, who died when I was a baby in a car accident, my mum remarried. From the moment he came into our lives he took me under his wing – and for this I am forever grateful. This experience has most certainly shaped my thinking into my adulthood and has played a big part in our decision to adopt.

I am looking forward to reading Will's workbook, and I wonder how much overlap there will be.

I have also been working on the paperwork I need for my overseas police check. The agency requires police checks for any extended stay in a country. For me, this would be for my travel to Vanuatu in the South Pacific. This seems an impossible task. After doing some research I have found out that yes, a police check can be done – slight problem though, the paperwork has to be hand-delivered to the police station in Port Vila, the capital. So unless the agency is going to be paying for a return flight, I doubt this is going to happen. I have suggested that as an alternative they ask for a reference from the organisation that I travelled with. Fingers crossed this will be satisfactory for them. Thank goodness no check is needed from India – my length of stays were shorter, so not required.

8 October

Our referees have now been asked to write our references. We have provided the names of six people, from close friends, family, our workplace and four additional people from places where we have volunteered. It is strange to think that these people are playing such an important role in our pathway to becoming parents.

Next week we are going on the training course. We are really looking forward to it. I have booked a lovely hotel in the centre of the town. It will be nice to get away and really concentrate on the course and not be distracted by travelling. We have both been given the three days off work, as part of our adoption allowance. I can't help wondering who else will be on the course. I really hope we make some friends through this shared experience.

15 October

We left early this morning for the hour and a half drive to the course venue. As expected we were a bit early, so sat in the café and had a coffee. While we were waiting we saw a panel meeting underway in one of the adjoining rooms. There was a couple waiting nervously; they were then called in. After about 20 minutes they emerged with what we imagined was their social worker, they hugged and cried – it was good news, how wonderful to see. Hopefully this will be us one day.

At the allocated time we entered the training room. We were the first couple to arrive and met the social worker who was leading the first session. After a few minutes a few other couples arrived. We all made a cup of tea, wrote our names on stickers and took a seat in the pre-formed semi-circle. Then entered a fourth couple. My immediate thought was, *'I think we will be friends'* – I just had a feeling we would have a connection with them.

The first task of the morning, an icebreaker, was to *'find out three facts about another person in the group, not the person you came with'.* I made direct eye contact with our potential new friend and made a beeline when we were asked to begin. I love these sorts of activities, Will less so. We shared a few facts about each other and found out we had more than adoption in common – we both love art and design. That's it, I am sure we will be friends. We had two hours of activities in the morning, lunch and then a further two in the afternoon. We began by learning about attachment, what it means to have secure attachments, how to develop attachment post-placement and insight into different types of attachment, and the impact of separation and loss on child development. We were then, using post-it notes, asked to write down our hopes and fears of adoption. These were anonymous and provided as discussion prompts in the following session. It was nice to see that others in the group had similar worries to us – ranging from loving someone else's child to not being selected to go through the process and the potential impact of trauma and abuse on child development. The social worker did her best to dispel any myths and put us at ease, saying that at this stage it is completely normal to have such worries.

The next session covered the different options for permanence in England and Wales, including adoption, Fostering for Adoption, Special Guardianship, birth parents, permanent long-term foster care or a child arrangement order.

I didn't realise there were so many variations of legal arrangements. For now we have been told that we will hear more about Fostering for Adoption on a future training day. Before lunch we watched a video, called the 'Still Face Experiment' (developed by Dr Edward Tronick in the 1970s). The video was used to highlight the importance of interaction, for developing secure attachments. It showed a toddler sitting in a highchair and a mother sitting in front, smiling and interacting. The mother used happy expressions to communicate, which prompted positive reactions from her baby. Then, for two minutes, the mother stared blankly, showing no emotion or interaction. It was hard to watch. The baby tried to make its mother smile by smiling, pointing, trying to get a reaction. After a short while, the baby got physically distressed by the emotionless mother; the aim of the experiment was to show the impact of non-emotional reactions on babies (Zero to Three, 2017 – for access to the video), emphasising the importance of attachment and interaction. After reflections from the group, we broke for lunch. As it was day one, most people chose to sit with their partner. Will and I didn't realise there was a canteen, so had come prepared. We tucked into our lunch and started to micro-analyse the session.

The next session was designed to get us to think about different types of attachment – secure and insecure – and the associated behaviours (including anxiety and anger). It was interesting and we were asked how we would cope with the different scenarios presented. I think 'cope' is an interesting way of framing it – I think any of us would try our best in the given scenario and do what we could to support the child with the resources and knowledge of the situation that we had at the time. It is so hard to know what you would do, until you are in the moment. The session really exposed us to some of the challenges associated with attachment. The final activity of the day focused on the grief that children experience when they are adopted. This was an excellent activity and I am sure that many of us will remember it for a very long time and reflect on it as we begin our lives with our children. The take-home message was *'children going through adoption will have experienced multiple losses before coming to you – they will be grieving.'* It was a role-play exercise. One of the participants acted as the child and stood in the centre and the rest formed a circle around her, each one acting as a key person in her life. We were all connected to the child with a piece of string. The social worker then read out the Child Permanence Report (CPR) and each time a connection was severed, the string was cut. As the extract continued the child had lost so many people in their life – from birth parents to grandparents, siblings, their allocated social worker, the health visitor, foster carer, teacher and their pets. By the end of the account, all connections had been severed; no connection with her past remained. This was a powerful activity to be involved in, a real eye-opener into the harsh realities for many of the children who are adopted.

The session ended at 3pm. We said our 'goodbyes' and 'see you tomorrows' then headed to our hotel and checked in for our stay. We are so glad that we made the decision to stay away for a few nights. We are tired and feel drained so went out for dinner then returned for an early night. There is so much to process but we are looking forward to tomorrow.

For a little more context I felt it was important to give some more background as to why children are adopted in the UK. The latest government figures (reporting period 2019–20) show that of the 3440 children adopted, abuse or neglect accounted for the majority at 77 per cent, family dysfunction 12 per cent, family in acute stress 5 per cent, parent's illness or disability 3 per cent, absent parenting 2 per cent, child's disability 0.5 per cent and socially unacceptable behaviour 0.5 per cent of cases. For a detailed review of all data on children adopted in the UK, see UK Government (2021).

16 October

Day 2 of training they said would be 'intense' and they were right. The focus of the morning was the impact of neglect, trauma and abuse on children and then in the afternoon, we learnt about therapeutic parenting and the importance of our support networks. By 9am we had all taken our seats, the same as yesterday, in a semi-circle in the training room. The social worker was surprised to see that we had all returned. It is common that not everyone will return on Day 2; sometimes up to 50 per cent of the group decide that adoption is not for them after the first day.

The activity on different forms of abuse was designed to encourage interaction with each other and to make us think about how we would cope with a child that had been exposed to different types of abuse – ranging from emotional, physical, sexual and neglect. Some in the group understandably found this session difficult; through our professional work, we were less shocked and more saddened. Impacts on children ranged from eating disorders, stealing food, low self-esteem, lying, self-harm, flashbacks, passive, aggressive, fearful, sleep issues, sexually inappropriate behaviour and negative impact on brain development. Abuse also happens in utero. We were told a shocking example of a baby who was removed at birth and placed in foster care. A few months into the placement the foster carers were pleased with her progress. However, during a visit to a fast-food restaurant, the baby became visibly distressed, inconsolable. They mentioned the incident to their social worker and were told that the birth mother had lived above one of these restaurants while pregnant. The birth mother was a victim of domestic violence and the impact on the baby through this incident became clear. The baby associated the smell in the fast-food restaurant with a time of stress and anxiety. The birth mother, experiencing an abusive relationship while pregnant, would have been in fight-or-flight mode – this would have released the stress hormone cortisol – known to have an impact on the development of the baby (Sandman and Davis, 2012). This example shocked the group. Here was a baby who was experiencing stress, not from the impact of drugs or alcohol, but from a stressful in utero experience.

The training then moved on to discuss different forms of contact (such as Letterbox contact) and ongoing relationships with birth parents. I will be honest, before the session, I wasn't sure this was something that we would be comfortable in doing. Now though I can see the value of Letterbox (an exchange of letters between the adoptive and birth family, often on a yearly basis) and other forms of contact, if appropriate for the child and the situation. We were shown evidence of the importance of Letterbox contact for encouraging a sense of self and security in children, adolescents and adults. On a future training day we will be shown examples of Letterbox communication, from both perspectives (adopters to birth parents and vice versa). At this stage it was time for lunch. Today we all ate together, sitting on a long table in the café. It was lovely to be able to speak to the other couples and compare notes.

The session after lunch began with another visually impactful activity, one that again I am likely to remember. It was called 'The Wall' (a representation of this can be seen at Adoption UK, 2015). First, we were all asked to write a word on a piece of A4 paper; the word needed to represent what every child needs to build a foundation of a secure, stable happy childhood – I wrote *routine*. We were then asked to place our word(s) on the floor. Together, they formed a wall of words, including food, safety, sleep, love and care. Next, the social worker read out an extract from a CPR. We were asked to remove words when it was clear that this was lacking from the child's life. By the end of the extract there were not many words remaining holding up the wall. There were two clear messages. First, one of the only words left on the wall was 'love'. Many of the children that end up in the care system are indeed loved by their birth parents, despite the situation which has caused them to be removed from their family. There are circumstances that mean that this isn't enough to keep the child safe. The second message, if you adopt a three year-old (for example), they may not have had cuddles or food, and they may not have been kept safe and secure, so you may need to parent them like they are a one year-old. For these young children, they need to go through the developmental stages they have missed out on. This was such a striking activity and really made us think about the impact of trauma on young children.

We ended the day with a focus on the PACE model. Coined by Dan Hughes (see Hughes, 2021), this is a way of therapeutically thinking and reacting to your child. P stands for *playfulness*; this encourages a playful way of interacting with children, thinking carefully about tone and body language. Next, the A stands for *acceptance*; this acknowledges that you accept your child for who they are, their whole story, their emotions, feelings and sensitivities. C is for *curiosity*, encouraging us to be curious about why the child may be responding in such a way. Instead of saying 'why did you do that?', this approach encourages a different way of responding, instead saying, 'I wonder why you felt you needed to do that'. Lastly, E is for *empathy*. Showing empathy reinforces to the child that their life and feelings are important and the parent will be there through the hard times. We enjoyed hearing about the PACE approach, it made sense to us and we can see how it will be a useful way of thinking and reacting when we have a child placed with us.

It is now the end of the second day. We are exhausted; it has been mentally draining. After the course we headed to the hotel, had a drink in the bar and went for an early dinner. We had a good debrief, talking through the challenges of the material we have covered today. We also had a discussion about what we feel is an elephant in the room, the names of children that are placed. It hasn't been covered and nobody has asked questions about it.

We are interested in hearing more about under what circumstances names can be changed, particularly with the Fostering for Adoption process. We are sure we are not going to be the first, or last, adopters who are anxious about what names their children may come with – names that they feel may not 'fit' with their family, and indeed grieving the names that they hoped that a future birth child may have had. Let's see if anyone mentions it tomorrow. For now, we are getting an early night, ready for our final day of training.

One of the take-home messages from our second day of training was that as a prospective adopter you will need a good support network around you – both before and after a child is placed with you. There is a lot of myth-busting happening around adoption in the UK at the moment – to encourage diverse families to consider adoption. Here Kristie, a single adopter to twins, reflects on the importance of her support network:

> My situation is a little different to other single adopters – I live with my mum. When she is not at work, I have a lot of support. My agency has always been sensitive to this and have offered support should I need it. During the assessment process I had to show that I had lots of people to rely on if my mum wasn't there to support me. I love being a single mummy to baby twins – no matter how tired I am it doesn't matter when you see them smile.
>
> (Kristie, single mummy, Early Permanence Placement, twins aged six weeks)

17 October

We woke up excited this morning, looking forward to the final day and hearing about EPPs, or rather Fostering for Adoption. We are so pleased that we have now met a group of people who are at the same stage as us. There is talk of setting up a messaging group to keep in touch; one of the other couples is going to co-ordinate it. It will be good to compare notes as we move through the process.

The first session of the day was on next steps, the assessment process, going to panel, the role of the Agency Decision Maker (ADM) and then a look at Link Maker. This is the nationwide database of profiles. If after three months a match with children associated with the agency has not been initiated then adopters are welcome to have access to the database to widen their search. It was good to have confirmation of the next phase of the process, to see where we are heading, the timings and what to expect. Before we broke for a coffee break a hand was raised and out came the question *'Can we change the name of a child that we adopt?'* – all eyes were on the leading social worker. As we predicted, this is frowned upon, not recommended or encouraged by social workers, judges and all those involved. What followed was an interesting discussion about identity and belonging and the importance of a name. Will and I were left feeling that we know what would be the right thing to do.

The final session of the morning was excellent. It was led by an adopter and her little girl. She told us about her journey to adopting her child and the challenges she has faced along the way. She was honest and open about their experiences of adoption. Her little girl has foetal alcohol syndrome (FAS) – the most extreme end of the foetal alcohol spectrum disorders (FASDs) (see NHS, 2021, for more information). They were aware of this diagnosis pre-adoption and spoke about the issues, such as the developmental delay that she is facing as a three year-old and what they are expecting in the future. Our agency stressed that it was important we understood the complications associated with FAS and the impact it can have, long term, on children's bodies and lives.

After lunch the focus turned to Fostering for Adoption. Aside from reading a few leaflets about this route to adoption, we were looking forward to learning more. In these cases the young child (often aged 0–2) is placed with potential adopters on a fostering placement, while the professionals collect evidence and the court ultimately decides on the outcome. The main emphasis of the discussion was about the risk and uncertainty which adopters take when agreeing to a Fostering for Adoption placement. There were lots of opportunities to ask questions about how it works in practice, what contact with birth parents can look like, the paperwork and fostering requirements and the likelihood of the 'baby going back' scenario – which I am sure is one of the most anxiety-inducing aspects of the process. At the end of the session a few of the couples in our group were interested in Fostering for Adoption. At this stage we were told to keep our options open; they advised that we work towards being approved for both traditional adoption and Fostering for Adoption. The training finished mid-afternoon, and we all exchanged numbers and said goodbye.

As we drove home, we reflected on the three days. It has been informative and interesting. We have become much more aware of the challenges associated with adoption, particularly trauma. It has made us think about our own childhoods and attachments. Both of us grew up surrounded by secure attachments; our lives were protected, consistent and predictable. It is good that at this stage we have been exposed to potential childhood traumas that we could be faced with.

Another early night for us, with three days off for the training. It's back to work tomorrow for a few busy days of catching up.

After the training we were excited by the potential of being able to bring home a baby on a Fostering for Adoption placement. As I explained, only a few couples in our training session felt it was something that they would want to do; it was considered too risky for most. In the case study below Jessica and Mark share their experience. Post-training and throughout the process, they had not planned to accept a child on this type of placement but once they 'got the call' and heard about the unborn twins, they knew this was a match for them.

> We hadn't planned to do Fostering for Adoption, or as our agency calls it, an Early Permanence Placement (EPP). We had attended the training session to keep our social worker happy and didn't expect to come out of the session agreeing that EPP may be an option for us. We knew that we wanted to adopt sibling boys we had read early on that siblings and boys are more difficult to place and this struck a chord with us. As we have two birth daughters (aged 14 and 11 at the time of our family deciding to pursue adoption), we felt sibling boys would fit nicely into our family dynamic. We had expected to be matched with a couple of toddlers and didn't think EPP would be relevant for two older children.
>
> We reached the end of Stage 2 during the Covid-19 lockdown and were a couple of months away from Adoption Panel when our social worker called. I was at work but answered and my battery was low. I remember her saying, 'You will want to be near a charger, this is a long conversation.' It turned out to be a really short conversation. She read me an early alert document detailing identical twin boys due to be born in two weeks. They were to be removed at birth and placed with EPP carers as the likely outcome for them was adoption. Our social worker told me to discuss it with my husband and come back with a decision the following day.

It's surprising, and scary, how little you know going into an EPP. As the children were not yet born, there is no CPR – it hasn't been written yet. The babies had no known health conditions but would be induced for a premature birth. The birth mother had tested positive for narcotics and suffered considerable domestic violence. We had a paragraph of information to make a decision that would affect the rest of our lives. We didn't know if they would be born healthy, healthy, if withdrawal was likely or if they were to need special care for prematurity. It turns out that we didn't need any more information – we felt like these babies, precious little twins, were a gift – for which we were grateful. We agreed to take them into our hearts and deal with whatever unknowns came our way. After all there are no guarantees with birth children.

(Jessica and Mark, Early Permanence Placement/
Foster to Adopt, twin boys, 12 days old)

2 November

We have had a busy few weeks completing our workbooks. They are nearly there, just a few more tweaks to do tomorrow. Today is another big day on the adoption front and I woke up feeling nervous. We had our medicals with the GP. On reflection, we didn't have anything to worry about. Our doctor was supportive and calming; he did as much as he could to reassure us that we should be fine, medically, to get through this part of the process. We were weighed and measured, had our blood pressure taken and our medical histories reviewed – he was thorough.

The doctor will submit the paperwork, it will be reviewed by an adoption medical adviser at the agency and then hopefully we will have positive news.

3 November

Today brings us to the end of Stage 1 – we have put so much time and energy into our paperwork. The information we have given will be used by our allocated social worker in Stage 2 as a basis for our meetings. We have spent hours poring over the questions and words we have used to describe ourselves, our families, our relationships and reasons for wanting to adopt.

Along with the PAR we were also asked to submit i) our financial accounts, documenting our monthly incomings and outgoings; ii) a pet survey, where we were asked about the personalities and habits of our chickens, cat and tortoise; and iii) a self-declaration home survey, a check-list to ensure our home is safe and liveable for a child. We still need to get the chimney swept, secure the bedroom windows and of course finish our major kitchen renovation before our home will be signed off.

At 9pm tonight we hit submit on the online portal. That was it, Stage 1 paperwork submitted.

4 November

I am sitting on a plane, travelling to Rotterdam for a business trip. I am feeling unsettled. I know I am tired because of the emotional investment we have put into our paperwork over the past few weeks. However, I know the real reason I am feeling jolted. The last time I made this trip I was pregnant, although I didn't know it at the time. Soon after the trip, just before Christmas, I miscarried our second baby. As the plane took off, a wave of emotion surfaced. I am sad about what has been and anxious about the new journey we are on.

11 November

Today has been an important day for our parents as they attended our agency 'Friends and family training'. Adopters are encouraged to invite those in their support network to a half-day training session designed specifically for family and friends. We had primed our parents and they were keen; it was lovely that they were all able to go together. We made a day of it and afterwards went for lunch. They found it informative and it mirrored much of what we had been told during our training – about the trauma and abuse of many children in the system and how as our family they can support us, through the process, during the early days of placement and in the future.

There were a few takeaway messages that as we reflected on as a family. The social workers emphasised the importance of relationship building and not committing to contact with future children if the contact wasn't then built on. For us this won't be a problem – we are very close to our parents and we are sure they will have the opportunity to build strong, lasting relationships.

Second, our parents were shocked about not being allowed to see us in the early days of placement; of course, they would want to be on hand to support us, but for attachment building, it is important that the child is settled and knows who is who in the early days. Of course, we are hoping that with a young baby, there may be some flexibility with this.

Given our preferred route to adoption, our parents were a little disappointed that there was minimal information about Fostering for Adoption. Despite this, our parents are cautiously excited about what is to come.

25 December

We have spent many Christmases dreaming that the next will be 'the one' – the one where we have a baby. Christmas last year was traumatic; days before we had our 12-week scan only to find no heartbeat. We went from pure elation that our years of trying for a baby had succeeded, to the darkest of days. This year it is different; we are now on our way to being parents. The process of adopting a child is long and complex, but unlike IVF, we feel it is more likely to end with a child joining our family. Yes, this is yet another Christmas without a baby, but perhaps it is our last.

Little one, we are waiting for you.

CHAPTER 3

EXPRESSING OUR STORY: THE HOME ASSESSMENT AND ADOPTION PANEL

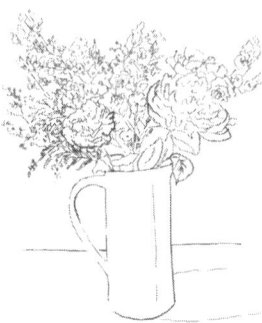

We begin this chapter with an air of optimism. Stage 2 ahead of us, there is hope that this will be the year that we become parents. Over several months we open our lives and hearts to our social worker, we ask critical questions of ourselves and question our expectations of parenthood. All of this work and emotional labour leads to our panel date, where a group of professionals decide if we, Alice and Will, are to become parents.

2019

1 January

It is the start of a new year and we have a spring in our step. We have got a busy few months ahead of us with our kitchen renovation starting in earnest this week and our first social worker visit for our Stage 2 assessment happening in the next few weeks.

8 January

The builders have started, as I type the floor is currently being dug out. Over the last few weekends, we have made a temporary kitchen and tried to keep the living room as normal as possible. Our social worker is visiting us next week, and I am panicking that she might take one look at the building work and ask us to put on hold Stage 2. Our builder is aware of how important the deadline is; we have just got to keep everything crossed there are no delays or problems.

16 January

Another big day. I now realise how many 'big days' there are in the adoption process, with each one feeling equally, if not more, important as the last. Today was the first meeting with our allocated social worker. We were nervous. We spent last night and the early hours of this morning cleaning and tidying.

She arrived at 10am on the dot. While we made cups of tea, she got out her laptop and paperwork. Our initial impressions were good. She seemed organised and professional. She opened with a compliment, saying that our workbooks were brilliant; she enjoyed reading them. This was so lovely to hear; we had put heart and soul into them. She explained that the focus of this first meeting was our experience of *'looking after, or working with, vulnerable young people'*. We felt comfortable and at ease as we answered her questions, drawing on quite a few examples of our volunteering and work experiences. She seemed pleased with our answers and was good at touch typing, writing notes on her laptop as we spoke.

We were honest and upfront about the situation with the kitchen renovation. She didn't have a look but we did tell her that it was major work being done – but importantly our deadline was Easter, which would be before the panel. She said that it shouldn't be a problem and she would leave our home inspection until our last meeting before the panel. As long as everything is done by then, it should be fine.

We had a chance to ask a few questions about the logistics of Fostering for Adoption – although she said that we would also learn more about this over the coming weeks. In terms of planning for the Stage 2 assessments, we asked if we could set dates for the next meetings. It is hard for us to work on a week-by-week basis as we need to organise our diaries a few weeks in advance. She was also keen on getting these booked, so we organised the next seven meetings. We really feel like we are making progress.

There were a few things that worried us. She asked us to imagine our future adopted child. In prompting us to think about this, she began by asking us to imagine our perfect child – *'have the image in your head, draw it on a piece of paper and throw it in the bin'* – this, she went on to say, is about lowering expectations. I have to say we were shocked and, after the meeting, quite upset by it. We really can't see why anyone would set out on a journey like this, adoption or otherwise, and have low expectations – why can't we hope and believe that this is going to be the perfect match for us? Yes, of course we know that the majority of children that come into the system have experienced trauma; this is part of them, today, tomorrow and always will be. However, we hope that if we are part of their story we can work together to find a better way, a way to go on, to live and to love. This child will be perfect to us, we will accept them for who they are.

We were also told about a few worrying cases of Fostering for Adoption. There was the example of a birth mother who breastfed her baby during the contact sessions. I was asked how I would feel about this. I have to say I was shocked. In my thinking through eventualities with Fostering for Adoption I hadn't considered that this might be a scenario that we could encounter. If we were forming attachments to a young baby, I am sure this would be difficult for us. However, the session encouraged us to flip our thinking – the point of contact with Fostering for Adoption is to maintain a relationship, so if the judge decides that returning to the birth family is in the best interests of the child a bond will be there. In this case, if breastfeeding is best for the baby, then this would need to stand. We were also told about a recent incident that happened during a contact session. The baby arrived at the contact session with a scratch on its hand; as a result, the birth mother made a formal allegation against the Fostering for Adoption carer. This upset me. My mind went into overdrive, thinking about the potential impact – on us as a family and our careers. At the end of the session she gave an overview of Care Orders, interim placement orders and something about the importance of '26 weeks' (we now know that court proceedings aim to conclude within this period – see Broadhurst et al (2018) for a detailed overview of the care proceedings surrounding newborns entering the care system in England) – I have to say all of this was a bit of a blur. I was still panicking about us potentially being accused of harming a baby.

Our meeting drew to a close after two hours and unfortunately Will had to dash back to work; we didn't even have five minutes for a quick chat. I was emotionally drained and couldn't stop thinking about the 'worse case' scenarios we were given. I know we are told about these cases to make us think and to challenge us, but I am not sure day one of our assessment was the best time. I know the social workers have to be honest, but it can be quite overwhelming.

Tonight our neighbours invited us for dinner. They offered to cook us a meal due to the state of our kitchen. It was good to be able to talk through our experience of the meeting and try to relax; it had been quite a day. We spent some time tonight reflecting on the 'throw it in the bin' comment – perhaps we may have taken this exercise to heart – with so much stress and pressure riding on these moments, I am sure some things get misinterpreted and taken out of context.

17 January

I woke up feeling anxious about potentially choosing the route of Fostering for Adoption. During the training we were told about the risks and emotions involved, with the main risk being that the baby can be returned to the birth family – but the other scenarios we were told about yesterday really jolted and scared me.

18 January

In the early hours of this morning I woke up and was upset. I had a nightmare. It was terrible and without a doubt prompted by our first visit a few days ago. I dreamt that Will and I went through all of this – we had done the training, the assessments, got through the panel, been matched with a baby – then Will died. This may seem extreme but it has been a reoccurring nightmare over the years, losing Will. This time though, with a tiny baby to care for, the nightmare was particularly terrible. There is no way I could do this on my own. We are a team, we need to do this together. This will be our baby.

Of course, I know where this stems from. My father died in a car accident when I was a baby. As I approach the same stage of life that my mum was, when she had me, I can't help but be anxious about this.

Today I also chatted with a close friend about the Fostering for Adoption scenarios we were presented with. We spoke about the potential for allegations to be made against us. She encouraged me to think about it in another way – this parent is going through the unimaginable, a child being removed from her care – she is doing anything possible, within her power to keep them. They need to do this.

During our training and assessment, the discussions about meeting birth parents were quite brief. We were not told very much about how contact with birth parents happens in practice – what is a contact centre like? Who is at the contact meetings? What risks are involved? This book shows a range of experiences of contact with the birth family (both positive and challenging). First, Charlotte and Richard reflect on their experience of contact with birth family where both of the children in their care had different contact arrangements. In their experience, the contact arrangements did not always go to plan.

> Our experience of contact with birth family was not as we expected. Our first contact session was in hospital before we were discharged, then all others at a contact centre with a duty social worker. After the first three contact sessions Little Brother was allocated his regular contact slots and contact workers. They were both lovely and we were comfortable leaving him under their supervision. We were however disappointed with the contact process. Little Brother's social worker had diligently outlined contact procedures but unfortunately these were not implemented by the first duty social worker – it was as if she hadn't even read the file. We were told that birth family would arrive 15 minutes before contact and wait 15 minutes before leaving, giving us the opportunity to arrive and leave – on numerous occasions I was putting Little Brother into the car and birth mother was in the car park. This was unexpected, stressful, and made us feel unprotected during a difficult time where birth family members behaviour may be unpredictable. On our first three visits, we were expected to hand Little Brother over in person to birth mother. We questioned this and were told that this should not have happened. This was the fault of the first duty social worker

who hadn't followed procedure and subsequent contact workers who then took the birth mum's word on the arrangement. As we are now into a routine of handing him over in person, we decided to maintain doing so – this was our decision. We felt that an opportunity had been created for us to hopefully establish a positive line of communication with the birth family.

From day one we used a notebook for any communication between us as the Fostering for Adoption carers and the birth family. We would write what had happened since the last contact visit and they would write details about their contact session. Before taking Little Brother to contact we would meticulously prepare the bag and pram for their visit, making sure they had everything they might need while ensuring that we didn't leave any personal items that might identify us. We had been told that birth family may bring their own items to contact; however, in our case sadly they never brought anything. I found this difficult to comprehend, particularly when I was criticised during one contact session for forgetting to pack the bottle of Infacol (for colic relief). On this occasion, I had stopped on the way (1.5 hour journey) to feed him and then forgot to put it back in the bag. I was so upset that this was commented on, particularly as the birth mum never brought anything to the contact sessions.

Contact would take most of the day because of the travel involved. We travelled to birth mother's area given that we needed to keep our location private (as we had Big Brother also in our care). The contact days were long and exhausting. One of us stayed with Big Brother at home, while the other took Little Brother to contact. If we had not been able to manage this, Little Brother would have been taken to contact by a social worker and the birth family would have needed to travel for contact.

As Fostering for Adoption parents we felt exposed in contact sessions and as a result found this process emotionally difficult to navigate. We had to be adaptable, resilient, work well with professionals and know that our expectations may not be met. Thankfully communication, both ways, has always been polite and respectful – we all wanted to build the best relationship possible given the difficult situation. We have been told that our relationship is as good as it gets and this is because of the interactions Fostering for Adoption created in our situation – we are grateful for this and believe it will only benefit us all and most importantly the boys going forward.

(Charlotte and Richard, Foster to Adopt, siblings, weeks apart, one from foster care and a baby from hospital)

From reading these case studies and speaking with other Fostering for Adoption parents who have had experience of contact, it can be hard. Not only are you learning how to live with a new baby but you may have to be travelling to contact sessions, several times a week. Here, Louise and Ian speak about the practicalities of contact, what they had to do in advance of each session and the reporting that went along with this:

We had a separate change bag for contact, as well as specific clothes that her birth parents had given her. We also included toys. Very quickly we were asked to prepare formula as the contact supervisors were concerned about hygiene. We wrote about events, milestones and activities in contact books before each session. We never had any written response and we don't know if the information we provided was read. We did get messages passed through the contact supervisors, such as she had the wrong nappy size (she didn't), missing gloves and she was always changed into her spare clothes.

(Louise and Ian, Foster to Adopt, girl, three months)

Contact with birth parents on a Fostering for Adoption placement can go on for months; it can be a long and exhausting process. In the case study below Rachel draws on her experience of contact with birth family over an extended period and the logistics involved. It was unsafe for her to take Jack to a contact centre, so he was escorted by a social worker. These were long journeys for Jack and this had an impact on him months after contact ended.

Jack attended contact with his birth family three times a week for nearly six months and this began a few days after he was placed. It wasn't safe for me to meet his birth family so I handed Jack to a contact supervisor who took him to and from the session each time. He found the travelling very stressful, even several months after contact had finished Jack was still unable to tolerate a long journey in the car, quickly becoming distressed and difficult to console. Over a year later this has settled but I don't think he will ever be choosing a road trip for fun. At seven months Jack's Placement Order was granted, he had a 'goodbye' contact session a few weeks later.

(Rachel, Foster to Adopt, boy, six weeks)

There are also Fostering for Adoption scenarios where a plan for contact with birth parents is not possible or recommended. In the case study below, Joanne and John reflect on their experience of accepting a relinquished baby where the birth parents did not want any contact post-placement. They acknowledge that while this made their Fostering for Adoption experience less hectic, they feel sad about this lack of contact for their little one.

> When birth mother found out that she was pregnant she decided that she wasn't able to care for her baby. She made the choice to relinquish her parental rights straight after birth and to have no contact with us or our little boy. We knew this soon after agreeing to the placement and although it made the first few months logistically easier, it makes my heart so sad. They have also chosen not to have Letterbox contact. However, we have decided to write once a year, in case, in the future, they change their minds.
>
> It feels strange to have never met the people who created such a joyful and smart little boy. I'm sad that they never met him and may never know how well he is doing and how handsome he is. I'm also sad that he will have so little information about his birth parents and the situation which led to them making the decision of adoption.
>
> (Joanne and John, Concurrent/Fostering for Adoption, boy, one day old)

19 January

Since beginning Stage 2, we have been telling more friends and family about our intention to adopt and their response has been overwhelmingly positive. It has been so lovely to have the support of our close network. However, a few people have thrown me off guard with their reaction. Today was one of those instances. I was in a meeting with a colleague and we were making plans for next year. I felt it was only fair to tell him that we were hoping that within the year I would be on Adoption Leave. He genuinely looked pleased to be able to say *'well we know exactly what that feels like, we recently adopted a dog'.* I was taken aback that he compared the process of adopting a baby to that of a dog – there was no sarcasm or joke to follow, he genuinely meant it. I smiled and quickly moved the conversation on. Inside I was raging; he has no idea what we are going through to grow our family.

20 January

It has almost been a week since our first social worker meeting and we are now gearing up for the second. The enormity of what we are doing and the risks that are involved have hit me – I have been emotional over the past few days thinking through the various scenarios and outcomes. Will keeps telling me that it is best not to overthink it. Let's try to keep calm and focused.

22 January

Our second home visit was this afternoon from 2 to 4pm. Our social worker had emailed us at the start of the week to say that the focus of our discussion was to be *Loss and Separation* – my first thought, '*in at the deep end again*'.

We sat in the same seats as last week, she opened her laptop and asked the first question. I had to stop her there. I couldn't quite believe I was about to say this. Will glanced at me in horror. I said, '*I am really sorry, but before we start on the topic for this week, would you mind if we could spend a few minutes reflecting on last week?*' I felt this was really important. I needed her to know that we had been scared by the Fostering for Adoption scenarios she had told us. We had felt drained and it had taken us the week to process the information and prepare for her second visit. She appreciated me saying this and she did what she could to put us at ease.

We then began with the questions and took it in turns to answer. Will spoke about the relationship he had with his grandparents and the impact that their deaths had on him. I then reflected on my father and grandpa dying and the miscarriages we had experienced. I also spoke about my granny who is living with dementia – a type of loss, a feeling of grief but with no death. She is physically with us but, in so many ways, not with us. This session was tough. I tried to hold back but big tears rolled down my cheeks. I have never thought about some of these questions, feelings and emotions, let alone spoken about them out loud.

She also asked us to reflect on grief during the adoption process. Adoptive parents may grieve for a biological child that they are unable to have; their children may also grieve for a fantasy child–parent relationship, something so magical that the reality will never match expectation. As we learnt during our training, adopted children will no doubt experience grief. There will be ties cut and relationships and attachments grieved. They will also experience a change in routine. This is a difficult transition process and as adoptive parents we need to understand this. More tears followed; this was emotional.

After the meeting Will and I were able to have a proper debrief session, without both of us dashing off to work. We said goodbye to the social worker, closed the door behind us and cuddled. We needed it. The session was tough; we were exhausted and drained but we definitely felt better than we did last week. I was happy that we addressed our anxieties at the beginning in the moment of reflection. This was important.

23 January

We woke up this morning feeling happy. We are getting good vibes from our social worker; we are going to like working with her. She seems fair, organised and honest.

I had a meeting today with my HR department about my plans for Adoption Leave. I felt it was important to be open about our intention to do Fostering for Adoption because for my employer and colleagues this is going to have significant implications. Due to the speed at which placement can happen, they and I need to be prepared for me to leave quickly. They were unaware about Fostering for Adoption but it seems that they are going to make sure it is covered in their adoption policy – a good sign.

25 January

Today was our final compulsory training session. The focus was post-adoption support, life story work, matching and Theraplay. Unfortunately, this was a different group of people from our Stage 1 training. It would have been nice to meet up with everyone again. This group were at different stages of the process. We were all asked to introduce ourselves and, in doing so, reflect on the origin of our name. This was it. This was the moment that they talk about names, identity and belonging. We have been told how important it is that children's names are not changed in the adoption process, unless for safeguarding reasons the name is too identifiable. The discussion which followed was a little awkward. Many in the room expressed anxiety over not being able to change a child's name – particularly young babies. However, the agency, social workers and courts are against name changes, to reduce the impact on the child. Of course, Will and I have discussed this; yes, we have always dreamt of choosing a name for a child. Indeed like many, we have some names in mind – however, as we learn more about adoption we are also sympathetic to the damage that changing a child's name can have on their identity and belonging.

Next came the life story session. This was interesting. The social workers explained that *'children who live with their birth parents have the opportunity to know about their past and have a means to being able to understand it. Children separated from their birth families are often denied this, they may have changed families, social workers, homes and neighbourhoods. Their past may be lost, much of it forgotten'* (taken from my notes). This is why life story work is so important. It is important for parents to discuss the past with their children; it is their story and theirs to understand. One of the session participants was herself adopted – it was amazing to hear her experiences and reflections on life story work. She was adopted at the age of one and has had a happy and full life with her parents. However, she has no information about her birth parents or foster carers. She said something which really struck a chord *'nobody in my life knows my full story.'* Her voice quivered and a tear was shed. This was the moment, the moment I knew that I wanted to do Fostering for Adoption. I want to know the full story of our little one, I want to be able to fill in the gaps and be there to share their story as they grow up.

We also heard about the significance of the Later Life letter. This is usually written from the child's social worker to the child, to explain the situation and professional decision making that led to adoption. This is a chronology of names, events and dates which hopefully would answer questions that the child may have when they are old enough to understand.

Before lunch we were told about 'next steps' post-panel. Every month there is a 'Matching and Tracking' meeting where social workers discuss the children awaiting a match and the pool of adopters who are approved. We were told that a child's social worker will read adopters' profiles and, if interested, will request the full Prospective Adopters Report (PAR). At this stage they may request to see two or three PARs; these will be shortlisted and the social worker will visit these families before making a decision on the placement. I don't think we had really appreciated the 'chosen' part of the selection process; I am now worrying that we might not get picked.

The afternoon session focused on 'Theraplay' – an interactive workshop which taught us how to use play techniques to support secure attachments. The activities focused on four key themes: structure, nurture, engagement and challenge, and primarily used touch through objects such as feathers and mimic. The purpose is to develop emotional connection and promote secure attachment, empathy, self-regulation and trusting relationships. We enjoyed the session and picked up a few new ways of communicating through play. I consider myself to be a playful person – so it looks like these skills will be useful one day.

This evening we had arranged to stay with Will's parents. We had a lovely evening talking about the session and what we had learnt. Now that we have completed the compulsory training, we have a clear pathway over the next few months, completing our home assessment, feedback on our PAR, panel and then to matching and tracking – exciting.

It was so interesting to learn about life story work in our training session. During the day we were able to see examples of best practice life story books – some were handmade, others professionally printed. Here Rachel speaks about the life story work she has done with her little boy. She emphasises how important it is for them as a family to have these conversations, so his story grows up with him:

> Although he is still very young I speak to Jack about his life story. I have made a simple version of his life story book into a baby board book so that he can handle it himself and look at the pictures and become familiar with who is who, in the hope that when he is old enough to look through his full life story book nothing will come as a major surprise to him. I want Jack to know that he is loved very much by both his family now and his birth family and that lots of people wanted to care for him.
>
> (Rachel, Foster to Adopt, boy, six weeks)

6 February

Today was our third social worker session; the topic 'our relationship'. Compared to previous topics, this seemed easier. We are a solid unit, work as a team, are happy and supportive of each other. At the end of our assessment process we will meet with our social worker individually. She explained that this is important – she has to check that couples are equally invested in the adoption process and there is no coercion.

Last session we were given a CPR to read; she wanted to know our thoughts and reflect on it in the session today. Prior to the meeting Will and I had read it independently and then discussed it. We talked about the chaotic nature of the family life which surrounded the child. It read like everyone in the scenario was struggling, from the birth parents to grandparents, aunts and uncles. We felt like some of this struggle came from the wider social and economic system and not being able to break the cycle, but on the other hand, there were serious mistakes and misjudgements on the part of the child's family. We were encouraged by the level of support that had been offered to the family and the chances they were given to improve their situation for the benefit of the child. We raised these points in the meeting and had a good discussion about it. Our social worker wanted to push us further. She wanted us to read it again and this time reflect on the behaviour of the child, the reasons behind this and importantly how we think we would cope caring for a child displaying characteristics such as violent or sexualised behaviour. We will address this next time.

Over the past few weeks Will and I have talked about our preference for a girl. I have always imagined having a little girl and Will (to my surprise) has quite a strong desire for a girl as well. However, we have decided that we don't think our social worker would appreciate us making this choice at this stage, so we decided to keep this to ourselves. Today we were asked directly about gender – we said we would be open to either. I am glad we had talked about this before today. She went on to say that she was not keen on adopters making a preference; she also said that some social workers actively move away from adopters who have specified gender. I think we need to be open-minded about this. What we do know is that we want to go down the Fostering for Adoption route. We want the chance to have a baby from a young age.

As we move through the assessment process I can feel the pressure increasing. I am feeling emotional thinking about how important this is to us.

At this stage in the process we had set our hearts on Fostering for Adoption. We wanted the chance to care for a baby as young as possible, preferably newborn. Most of the examples we had heard about in our training had been about newborn babies being placed from birth. In the case study below, Charlotte and Richard share their experience. They were placed with a child and a month later the Little Brother was born; this was a sibling placement. Charlotte shares her detailed experience of being there from the very beginning for 'Little Brother' – for her, totally amazing and a privilege to be able to bond from day one:

> Big Brother had been living with us for just over a month when his little brother was born. We got a text message (over the weekend) to say he had been born, the time, his weight and when the midwife thought he would be ready to be discharged. On the Monday his social worker went to court and an Interim Care Order was granted. She asked if one of us could go to the hospital to be with him as his birth mum had chosen to leave after news of the court decision, rather than staying with him in hospital until he was ready to be had been meticulously prepared to collect him from the hospital at a moment's notice but I hadn't packed a bag for myself so I quickly ran upstairs and was out the door and en route in ten minutes. Driving to the hospital I rang my mother and best friend. I was excited and nervous, how would I know what to do? No one lets you look after a newborn baby to practise. I met his social worker in the hospital foyer and we went up to the Special Care Baby Unit. I met him for the first time; he was fast asleep in his crib and his social worker picked him up and handed him to me. She said she couldn't imagine what I had been through to get to this point. She didn't stay long and we were left together on the ward.
>
> The nurses were amazing and so supportive; they treated me like a new mother and wanted to provide the experience and support that a mother who had given birth would have. The ward sister fed him and showed me what to do. Given that it was getting late she suggested that I get some sleep – she would wake me to do the next feed and observe. If she was happy and I felt confident then he could be moved from the ward into the private room with me. This was the most amazing feeling

and a reality I had accepted I wouldn't experience – caring for a newborn baby in hospital was a time I will treasure. Having the joy of sleepless nights, feeding and winding a baby because he was my responsibility to care for and protect was a dream come true. I couldn't believe how calm and content he was. This time together was so precious and felt so peaceful. I was surprised to find how natural everything felt and the instant connection I felt for this baby. The team were happy for us to stay for as many days as we needed to settle in together but the next day I knew we were ready and the ward sister felt the same.

Before we could leave there needed to be a Discharge Placement Meeting with his birth mother, his social worker, the ward sister and myself to discuss his care. Prior to this meeting we had met the birth mother once during introductions with Big Brother. We had been told that she liked us and showed obvious relief at finding out that Little Brother was also being placed in our care. However, I don't think she really understood or realised that adoption may be the most likely outcome for her baby at this time.

Our interactions have always been polite and respectful; she has however always presented as emotionally withdrawn. After the meeting a contact session with Little Brother and birth mother was scheduled. I handed him over and his social worker observed the session. Once contact was finished he had a feed, we collected our belongings and left to go home.

Given that Big Brother had only recently been placed with us, he and my husband didn't get to meet Little Brother for two days. Big Brother could not be left in the care of anyone else and them coming to the hospital posed a risk. The birth mother had the right to return to the ward at any point until Little Brother was discharged – if my husband and Big Brother were visiting and the birth mother turned up, this could have potentially been very damaging to the attachment we were building with Big Brother.

They both greeted me at the door when we arrived home; it was so special. Like me, my husband felt that caring for a newborn came naturally. Obviously he had seen photographs but he couldn't believe how tiny he was; he was on the 2nd percentile and so fragile. We had a week to settle in as just the four of us before contact began the week after. We chose to live in the present and focus on the amazing moments of seeing a baby grow and develop from birth. We knew the risks we had taken by saying yes to a Fostering for Adoption placement but we were committed to caring for him and loving him as though we would be his parents forever.

(Charlotte and Richard, Foster to Adopt, siblings, weeks apart, one from foster care and a baby from hospital)

Similar to Charlotte and Richard, Beatrix and Thomas also accepted a sibling placement, with one child being 22 months and the other newborn. In the case study below they share their experience of a quick match after the Adoption Panel and the whirlwind of a week as two children, under two, moved into their home:

Two under two, that is what we wanted from the beginning. We had been through IVF and miscarriages; we felt like we had to take the risk. A couple of days after panel we got a phone call; we were getting ready to go out for lunch and a call came through from the Family Finder. They said the next day they were going to be in court with a little girl, a few days old and her older brother. Almost immediately we agreed, *'we will do it'*. We went into work the next day and after a few hours we got a call to ask us to go to hospital to pick up the baby girl. We knew straight away that these were going to be the babies for us. We had seen no profile, no photos, just baby S and baby K; other than a brief verbal scenario, that is all we had to go on.

The drive up to the hospital was nerve racking. Her birth parents wanted to meet us in the hospital. It was tense. We walked into the room, birth mother stared at Beatrix, she handed the baby to the midwife and stormed out. Birth father stayed and thanked us. It was all over in ten minutes. Before we knew it, we were sitting in the car, looking in the mirror at the tiny baby in the car seat. This was the start. The next day we met baby K and after a few days of transition he came home. It was all systems go. Beatrix's mother came round and started washing baby clothes that our friends had dropped off, all our friends offered help which was amazing. By Monday evening we were sat with a baby in our arms and a little one sleeping upstairs. We had two beautiful children in our care, it had all happened so quickly, it was tough.

(Beatrix and Thomas, Foster to Adopt, S five days old, K 22 months, siblings)

9 March

It was the annual family gathering today. With Will's dad being one of nine, we have a large family. There are now over 30 grandchildren and great-grandchildren. Hopefully next year there will be another little one added to the family ranks. I really hope so – we can't wait to spend special days like this together.

10 March

I have had that wonderful nesting feeling today. I want everything 'just right' for when our little one arrives. We sorted drawers and cupboards and started to feel like we are getting ready for a child to join us.

24 March

We have just returned from a weekend camping and cycling in Wales with some of our neighbours. It was brilliant, a much-needed trip to unwind and destress. We had a lovely surprise when we returned home: the kitchen units have arrived, and they look beautiful. It is now all starting to come together – I am now more optimistic that we will have a fully functioning kitchen by the time of our home assessment.

26 March

Tomorrow is my individual assessment and our social worker has told us that I needed to have all of our finances ready to go through. It is a bit ironic that she is doing this with me as Will is the one who sorts out all of the paperwork. We put a few hours aside this afternoon to go through the folder that Will has prepared; let's just hope I can answer all of her questions.

27 March

I felt quite nervous about doing a session on my own. What if I say the wrong thing? Mess it up for both of us? As usual I was up early to make sure the house was tidy. The kitchen renovation is now in full swing and at the stage where it looks its worst. The social worker hasn't actually asked to see it yet – everything is happening behind a plastic screen. Today while we were sitting in the living room chatting, there was the loudest and longest drill making its way through one of our thick walls. She definitely knows it is happening.

We started by talking about the volunteering work that I had done with children and young people – there were a few more details she needed for our PAR. She then asked to look at our finances. My heart went in my mouth. I was nervous. She then admitted that mathematics and finances were her weak point, at which point I laughed and said 'me too'. I pulled out Will's very organised and labelled folder containing all our standing orders, money in the different accounts, incomings and outgoings – she was impressed with the level of detail. During our chat through the finances she didn't really give anything away – I think all was fine.

She then asked me more about our wishes for a little one, about potential ages, our interest in Fostering for Adoption, my feelings about not having a biological child and how we might deal with a situation where the baby has to go back to the birth family. Of course, this is one of the most anxiety-inducing aspects of Fostering for Adoption but we have talked about this a lot and Will and I both feel that it is a risk worth taking. We will welcome a baby into our home and if the unimaginable happens, then we will have to deal with the heartbreak and loss but be happy that we were able to be part of their life for however long it may have been for. I don't think you can think about it any other way.

There were a few activities that she did to prompt conversation about societal expectation of families. We had an interesting discussion about what a 'family' looks like and how society expects a family to look or behave. She then moved on to ask for a 'Pen Picture'; 300–500 words summarising us as a couple with a photograph. This is what children's social workers see when searching for adopters. This profile matters.

She was also keen to know what our parents might think about us accepting a baby who may be withdrawing from drugs. A difficult question to answer but one which I think is important. Our parents are an integral part of this process as ultimately they will be supporting us in the decisions that we make at the matching stage.

She ended the meeting by asking (again) if we were using contraception, and I told her, yes, we are.

31 March

Mothering Sunday. A day that is always tough for those who have lost babies and are in limbo, waiting to become parents. This Mothering Sunday is different. I am filled with hope and expectation, the hope that our baby is out there and this year we will meet them.

3 April

Another week has passed; I can't believe it. Today was our next session; we are coming to the end of the assessment. The session started with a discussion about the PACE model. We went through each of the aspects in turn, Playfulness, Acceptance, Curiosity and Empathy, showing what we understood is meant by them and how we might engage with it. Will and I do have a little giggle about the PACE acronym; for some reason Will cannot remember what it stands for. Occasionally, out of the blue, I will ask him and he comes up with other nouns, which sound reasonable but aren't actually PACE – we are working on it.

The discussion then moved on to focus on the relationship that we had with other family members. I was quite taken aback by the question *'Did your dad's family accept you as a child?'* I have never been asked this before and it has never crossed my mind. We are a family. I wasn't really sure how to answer the question, other than by saying *'yes, of course'*.

Today we also had to confirm which of our friends (also referees) would be willing to take on our child if both of us died. We were asked this via email a few weeks ago, which meant we had the conversation with our friends. Of course we very much hope that this would not happen, but it is a requirement of the process that we name them. We are very grateful that they are willing to do this; we know our baby would be safe, loved and happy if anything were to happen to us.

Towards the end of the session we were asked about our feelings towards direct contact with the birth family. We said that it was difficult to give our perspective on a situation that we have not yet been presented with. Of course, we would be guided by the professionals in terms of what would be in the best interests of the child. Until we are in that situation, we just don't know what we would do. We were told that judges are increasingly requesting ongoing direct contact as an arrangement post-adoption.

We ended with a walk around the house. She needed to make sure that we had worked our way through the checklist of jobs that needed doing – sweep the chimney, check; fit the window latches, check; buy two fire guards, check. The kitchen is a few weeks from completion, she can tell from the progress that has been made that it will be finished. She is happy that all requirements have been met. This is a big relief. We are nearly there; our house is just about ready to accept a child.

4 April

Tonight we sat down and wrote our 'Pen Picture'. It is hard to get the right tone. To be honest, I think we were overthinking it. It is also difficult to know which photograph to choose, how we want to be seen by a social worker that is potentially choosing our profile. We went with one of our holiday photographs in which we look relaxed and happy. We have drafted the statement and emailed it to our social worker for comments.

5 April

In advance of our next social worker meeting, we have been given what can only be described as a 'tick list' of variables to think through. We have to ask ourselves if we would accept a baby with heart problems; withdrawing from heroin; with a family history of schizophrenia; with hearing loss; the list goes on. I am so glad we have been given this in advance; we spent the evening going through each of these and doing some research on long-term impacts and the medical and social needs associated with each of the conditions. We have tried to be as honest as we can, although it is so difficult to think about.

Deciding to do Fostering for Adoption is a deeply personal decision. Adopters all come with their own stories and experience which undoubtedly shape their willingness to 'take the risk'. In the case study below Nicole and Paulo weigh up their feelings about Fostering for Adoption – given the long journey they have been on and the loss they have experienced on the way, the fear of potentially 'losing another baby' may be too much for them.

> We have been thinking about doing Fostering for Adoption for some time. When we began the adoption process over five years ago we had only recently lost our last pregnancy, our seventh baby. Fostering for Adoption felt too risky for us, we couldn't bear the thought of losing another. I am already in my 40s and have lost what feels like at least 15 years of motherhood.
>
> We are now drawing to the end of our Stage 2 assessment. Fostering for Adoption is still an option, but we may go down the traditional route. I still have the fear of losing another child if the court believes they should go back to their birth family. I don't think I have the strength to go through that kind of loss an eighth time. Paulo also has reservations; he had to live with a broken, grieving me for such a long time. Once we have done the Early Permanence training we will have to think about it carefully and talk it through with our social worker.
>
> (Nicole and Paulo, currently in Stage 2, considering Fostering for Adoption)

10 April

Today we had our last assessment session, focusing on children's profiles – it was a tricky conversation. I am glad we had the chance to think and talk through '*the matching tick list*' prior to the meeting. We went through each of the profiles, explaining our decision, hopes, expectations and anxieties. Our social worker was very clear that the backgrounds and trauma that even tiny babies have been through is more often than not extreme – that is why they are in the system. We actually found ourselves saying 'yes' to more conditions once we had discussed them with the social worker, and of course, most conditions have a sliding scale of severity (ie eye condition, which could mean wearing glasses to being registered as blind).

This is so abstract and hypothetical – until we hear about real children, real scenarios, we don't know what we will accept. She told us about a couple she worked with a few years ago. A baby had been born with a serious medical condition, the prognosis was poor, and it was likely that the baby would not survive days or weeks. There was one couple on the agency's register that they knew would accept the baby. They rang them and immediately they said yes. They were at the hospital a few hours later. The baby did survive and is doing really well, now aged two. This made us feel slightly awkward, as we can't imagine being in a position to accept a baby with such needs. As I said, we will have to see what profiles we are offered and we will have to weigh up the risks based on the information we are presented with.

We then went through the next steps. In her words she said there are *'lots of Fostering for Adoption babies at the moment'*, so it could happen quickly once we are approved. She then asked us if we would accept a six-month-old baby. I had a sudden pang of grief, a realisation that we may not be matched with the newborn that we desperately want. We will have to wait and see what happens, there are so many scenarios to consider – and that is if we even get chosen by the baby's social worker. She ended by saying, *'it might be quick or it may take up to a year'* – again another pang of sadness; how will we get through another whole year of waiting? The final step was to check our Pen Profile picture. She was happy with it and commented on our choice of photograph, and she said we came across as a *'relaxed, but fun couple'*. Post-panel she will upload it on the system for the children's social workers to see.

That is it then, the end of our home assessment. What an intense, whirlwind it has been. Every inch of our lives have been scrutinised – our relationship with one another, our family and friends, what makes us tick, what makes us upset, angry and happy. There have been questions I have never thought about before, questions no one has ever asked me. I have often felt like it has been like some sort of counselling, with an air of judgement thrown in for good measure. There have been tears, but also smiles and laughs – the whole spectrum of emotions.

21 April

The last few weeks have flown by and I realise I haven't written an entry. Since our last assessment we have been busy at work and at home. We are now on holiday and as I write I am sitting in our tent on the Isle of Skye looking out to the ocean. It is beautiful. We are a few days in to our time away and all we can do is hope that everything will be okay. We have done all we can do. We have opened our lives, our hearts and our home to our social worker; now we wait for her to finalise our PAR. It isn't long before we go to the panel, only a matter of weeks. Potentially any time after the panel (with the obvious caveat of being approved) we could be matched with a Fostering for Adoption placement – exciting and scary rolled into one. We keep saying that this might be our last holiday as a couple, I really do hope so. We are so ready to be parents, it must be our turn soon. For now though, we will eat lovely food, camp, go on long walks and keep everything crossed as we move into the next phase of the process.

Some adopters already have birth children. For these families there is much to do to prepare them for a new arrival, particularly when accepting a Fostering for Adoption placement. In the case study below, Jessica and Mark tell us about their experience of involving their girls in the decision to accept twins. In this case, their girls were old enough to understand that there was the potential for risk and the babies may only stay with their family for a few months:

> We have two birth daughters; they are both in high school and we fully involved them in our decision to adopt, right from the start of the process. We'd previously explained what Early Permanence Placement was, but that was all theoretical, until we told them about the twins. Our girls were in no doubt that we needed to say yes to these boys. We made sure they knew that we may end up just caring for these babies for a few months, and then would say goodbye. We all agreed that we would give them the best first few months as possible and deal with the heartbreak later if it came to that. We said that we would love the babies as if they were already 'ours' as they deserve that. I emailed our social worker that night to tell her yes, please proceed, we feel like we're the perfect family for these children.
>
> (Jessica and Mark, Early Permanence Placement/ Foster to Adopt, twin boys, 12 days old)

28 April

We arrived back home late last night and in our inbox was an email from our social worker. It was our PAR; she asked us to check and edit for any mistakes or irregularities. We made a cup of tea, nervously opened the document and made a start. It took us a few hours to go through it in detail. We are very happy with how we have been portrayed. There are only a few negatives (if you can really call them that). The first is that we haven't had any experience of caring for a baby overnight – although I can't really see how many people would have this. The other negative which we were aware of, which has been voiced as a concern at various stages throughout the assessment, is that we could be perceived by the panel as being too high achieving with too high expectations for a future child. If I am honest, this has upset us.

30 April

This is the busiest time of year at work. I really want to get on top of everything before our panel date. We have been told that Fostering for Adoption placements can happen quickly, without much warning. I want to make sure all my urgent work tasks are complete. I am starting a 'handover notes' file, which I will be able to pass on when the time comes for me to leave.

1 May

Boom. My first pre-panel meltdown, it hit me like a ton of bricks. I really thought I was fine and calm about our forthcoming big day, but clearly not. I am exhausted and working hard to get everything done; the pressure is really building. I have fear rising inside me: what if the panel decide that adoption is not for us, that we can't be parents? I can't bear to think about it.

5 May

For the last few days we have been staying in Durham, attending a friend's wedding. It was wonderful. We rented an apartment with my parents; a lovely treat before the panel. This afternoon we ended up practising answers to mock questions; I am feeling quite calm at the moment.

9 May

Prompted by thinking through the mock panel questions, today we decided to make some notes on themes we may get asked about. I thought it would be useful to share these here. This is our reality; this is what we are thinking through, the day before we go to the panel.

The process – on reflection we would say that it has been interesting, encouraging and professional. Fortunately we haven't had any hiccups or delays and we have been impressed with the social workers and their professionalism. I always think I am hypercritical, so for me to be impressed is very positive. We also think the process has been clear in terms of what happens next and expectation management. Of course, it has also been a steep learning curve. We have learnt about so many different aspects of adoption from attachment to the legal process and a great deal about ourselves. Since we started the process, our attitude and outlook have changed on a range of issues from the impact of trauma to being open about potential contact with birth parents.

Direct contact – we have been told that panels, and increasingly judges, are favouring ongoing direct contact (if it is safe and in the best interests of the child). Contact is increasingly seen as something that shouldn't be static and should be reviewed as the child grows up. Our social worker has prepared us for potentially having a child that has a plan for direct contact.

Our careers and apparent success – as this was raised as a potential point which the panel may want to push us on – what would we do if we had a child who wasn't 'academic'? If we are honest, we feel quite upset by this judgement. Yes, we have worked hard on our careers; however, we would say we would be sympathetic to a child's learning pace and style. We would play to their strengths, they would be given lots of opportunities, and we would be supportive and empathetic to their abilities. They will be who they'll be, and we will support them every step of the way.

Change in lifestyle – we imagine we may get a question about how our lifestyle will change and how we will cope with this. For us, our lives are busy and full because we have a child-shaped hole to fill. We will speak about being flexible and organised and the importance of our support network.

Attachment – we may get asked what we understand by attachment. It depends on the type of question, but I imagine that we would talk about going slow, PACE, working together, having a break and talking to each other about the challenges which we are facing. Let's just hope they don't ask Will what PACE stands for.

Understanding of Fostering for Adoption – we are pretty sure we will get a question about Fostering for Adoption as this is our preferred route. We will have to show that we understand that this process is risky. It is a route that is in the best interests of the child and us as the adopters will be taking the weight of the unpredictability and uncertainty.

Secondary trauma – there may also be questions about the impact of abuse and trauma on babies and children. There are some good examples from the training that we can draw on and we would emphasise that we would seek to understand the underlying cause of behaviour and any potential triggers.

Since getting home from Durham, my anxiety levels are increasing. In a panic I decided to have a look for some *'reasons why people are not approved as adopters'* – explanations ranged from the panel not agreeing that you are ready to adopt; poor references from your workplace, friends or family; inconsistencies in your application; to you having a medical condition that the panel believes would be problematic with a child in your care. I felt somewhat reassured but also scared by reading these reasons.

Tomorrow, a panel of people who we have never met are going to decide if we can be parents. The thought of that is quite overwhelming. Tonight, we have had a stream of texts from our friends and family, everyone is rooting for us. One text in particular made me smile: *'if you pair don't get through panel, I am heading out to buy the largest vat of superglue I can find and will stick myself to the council offices.'*

This is why you need your friends around you when you are going through the adoption process.

10 May

Panel day. This is what we have been building up to for all these months. I woke up in a bit of a mess; to be more precise it was a meltdown over what scarf I was going to wear. I had sorted my outfit last night, but not my scarf. I was wearing a navy dress, one of my favourites. The scarf, however, was a different matter. Does this one make me look fun? What about this one, too serious? A kind mummy? Too professional? The list was endless, so stressful, clearly I was overthinking it. A message from a friend put me at ease:

> *All of your scarves are lovely. I don't think they can read messages into a scarf. I am sure whatever you've chosen says 'I care about this meeting' and that is the main thing ... you are both going to blow them away.*

I selected a pink scarf and we made our way into town. It was a beautiful day, the sun was shining, and there were positive vibes in the air.

We had planned to be early, to give us time to potter. We had a look around a few antique shops (one of our favourite past times), had coffee in the sunshine and went over our notes. Just before we walked down to the council office we popped into a book shop. Will turned to me and said, '*We will have to bring him in here to buy a book.*' It was a little slip; he had said 'him' – very strange as we have only talked about having a girl. I don't think he realised he had said it. This sentiment really touched me; a moment I will never forget.

As we were walking towards the council office we were saying to each other that we didn't think we could be any more prepared. Then, out of nowhere, I had a sudden panic. I didn't know what *CoramBAAF* was – was it a government agency? A quango? A charity? I just felt I needed to know. A few quick Google searches were done en route, that base was covered. I could answer a question on CoramBAAF (it is a membership organisation for anyone involved in fostering or adoption). We waited for a few minutes in Reception, messaged our social worker to say we had arrived and were shown to a small meeting room. Nervous is an understatement. Our social worker came to us and almost immediately, as if a bit nervous, asked us if we were still taking contraception. Not something I expected her to say just before the panel but I imagine it does happen, couples conceiving naturally just before major decisions are made in the adoption process.

After a short wait, the Chair of the panel arrived. He introduced himself and said *'when you are ready, we are.'* Our panel slot was 11:40am; we followed him into the meeting room. The panel were sitting in a horseshoe, all eyes were on us. We sat down, took off our coats and opened our notebooks. We were ready. The Chair then asked for introductions. One by one the panel introduced themselves. I managed to scribble down the positions. We had nine attending: two independent foster carers, a social worker student, a social worker manager from the agency, a medical adviser, our social worker, the Chair, the Secretary and an adopter who was also a retired police officer.

We were told that there would be six questions, each one asked by a different member of the panel. Our questions were: i) how have you found the process? ii) how will you handle the fostering? iii) talk about how you would manage a non-academic child; iv) what medical needs might a child of 0–2 years have? v) what are you most looking forward to; and vi) any questions or queries?

We felt that we answered the questions well and both gave each other the opportunity to speak. Fortunately we had prepared for most of these questions, so there were no surprises. The medical question confused me slightly as I wasn't really sure what they wanted us to say. I thought it might be about the potential risk with a Fostering for Adoption baby and not knowing the full medical history at placement, so I spoke a bit about dealing with situations as they emerge. Will also said we had done research on FASDs and the potential impacts of drugs on unborn babies.

In answer to the question about what we were most looking forward to, I told the panel what had happened just before our meeting, in the bookshop. This is what I said I am most looking forward to, doing things together, the small, everyday things that make up a family and childhood. By this point I was crying, the tears had started. I had wondered if I would cry, sure enough this question did it for me. Will passed me a tissue and we moved on.

At the end of the questioning we were thanked and asked to leave the room. Our social worker stayed with the panel to answer a few more questions. We didn't have long to wait before we were called back into the room. We sat down and the Chair, with a beaming smile said, *'It was a unanimous decision, the panel want to recommend you for approval to the ADM.'* I glanced across the table and the ex-police officer winked at me. The next few moments were a blur with everyone expressing their congratulations. We had the approval of the panel. They were recommending that we could be parents – the best feeling in the world.

17 May

It has now been a week since our panel day and we are awaiting our final ADM decision, the stamp of approval for us to progress to the matching phase. We have now entered the phase of the unknown and I am beginning to feel it already. Next month, mid-June I am meant to be going to Norway for a few days for work. I have made the hard decision not to go. It is too risky, in case we get 'the call'. I had held off booking my flights but have now had a discussion with colleagues and have decided that I will join online. Being offered a baby with me being out of the country does not bear thinking about.

This afternoon we were given access to the online portal of children within our agency who are waiting to be adopted. Most of the children on the system are older than two and most are in sibling groups. We have read through the profiles but as our inclination is towards Fostering for Adoption, we were not drawn to any of them at the moment.

In the case study below, Jessica and Mark talk through their experiences of being matched with unborn twins who came to them on a Fostering for Adoption placement. Despite the process being quick and emotional, they felt this was best for them and the babies. During our training and preparation for Fostering for Adoption, we were told to expect a call to say that a baby was about to be born. For Jessica and Mark, this is what happened to them. This is their story:

> The next few days were a bit of a blur; we had telephone meeting with the family finder and a linking meeting by video with the children's social worker. There were then several phone calls back and forth from the agency as they tried to pull our Adoption Panel forward to the following week. We were told that the babies were being induced at the weekend but we wouldn't hear if they were even born safely until the following week – an incredibly difficult concept to accept. 'Our' children were to be born, and we weren't to be informed; we wouldn't know details of their birth, weights, health, or even names. This was the most difficult part of the process, the unknown. Our

social worker had said not to say anything to our friends and family until we were approved, and they had an Interim Care Order, but this is easier said than done – we had no baby equipment at all. I set up an Amazon shopping basket and started writing lists. We told our mums, and no one else. We just didn't know how the next couple of weeks would pan out.

We were linked the day before the boys were born, with panel a week later and we collected them a couple of days after that, at 12 days old. Birth mother, as expected, had requested a Mother and Baby Unit but this was turned down; she did not stay to care for the babies. They were fit and well, good weights given their prematurity, and they were moved from Special Care to Transitional Care quickly. The hospital were unable to keep them longer for us so they went to a temporary foster carer to wait for our approval to come through. I sent videos of us singing nursery rhymes and recorded reading stories for the foster carer to play them. My mum cried when I showed her the video.

I struggled this week. I cried, a lot. I was thankfully busy at work, with only a week's notice to get ready for Adoption Leave. I practised yoga, attended an online church sermon and prayed for these babies. When I see stories of traditional adoption, when the parents have known about their little ones for weeks, sometimes months, before bringing them home, I'm grateful for the EPP route. I am glad that our boys didn't have to go into longer-term foster care placements, waiting with someone else, waiting for the legal process to catch up so life in their forever family can start.

We had one visit to the foster carer and collected the boys the next day. Their tiny frames were swamped in new knitted hats and booties from an excited grandma. We came home to tears of joy from our daughters as they met their tiny new siblings for the first time. It was magical, and very personal. We hadn't 'gone public' with our new arrivals – only close family knew.

The following weeks were joyful and very busy with regular contact from a range of professionals including our social worker, their social worker, the health visitor, midwife, paediatrician, the children's guardian and the independent reviewing officer – all were supportive of the placement.

(Jessica and Mark, Early Permanence Placement/
Foster to Adopt, twin boys, 12 days old)

19 May

Today was an exciting day. We purchased our pram and car seat. There has been quite a build-up to buying these big-ticket items – it is scary to have to emotionally and financially commit to making these large purchases when we have no idea how our story is going to end. We have had our eye on them for some time and decided that today would be the day. Realistically we are only going to accept a baby under the age of six months, so we thought it was worth the risk buying the pram. The salesperson in the shop was brilliant, so excited for us and said the 'right' things about adoption and our journey to becoming parents.

In the afternoon I was a little overwhelmed. Our neighbours have been itching to hand over some baby clothes they have been saving for us. I thought they might give us a few items to borrow – well, I now think we need an extension. We sat on their spare bed and they brought out bag after bag after bag – they have been so generous. We are pretty much kitted out, we just need a baby now. It was overwhelming; we have waited for this for so long, now it is happening.

20 May

We saw my parents today and we were given two very special gifts. The first is a quilt that my mum has made for a future little one. It is beautiful, love has been sewn into every stitch. She also gave me the cot mobile that I had when I was a baby. My granny bought it for me and I had no idea that my mum had kept it for my future baby. This afternoon we hung it above the cot – it is perfect.

CHAPTER 4

WHO WILL JOIN OUR STORY? MATCHING, TRACKING AND AN EMOTIONAL ROLLERCOASTER

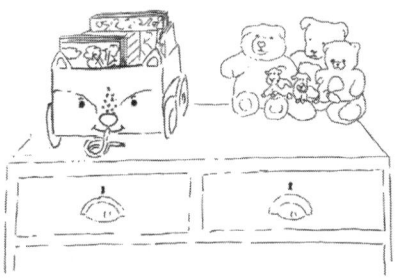

This chapter documents what for us was the hardest and most emotional stage of our journey to adoption. It is common to hear that the 'waiting' is the most difficult phase. Yes, we found it tough but it was this combined with the anxiety of making such a life-changing decision, the uncertainties and the process of Fostering for Adoption. Over many months we were emotional and stressed – but we now know that we had to go through this to get to where we are today.

22 May

We have had such a lovely time celebrating with our family and friends. Having a 'unanimous yes' has given us licence to start getting excited, get the nursery ready and buy some items for a future baby. The agency 'Matching and Tracking' meetings are monthly; our social worker emailed a few days ago to say she will be attending the next one on our behalf.

Well today was that day, the meeting was scheduled for the afternoon. We expected that we might receive an email tomorrow (throughout this process we find ourselves trying to pre-empt when we might get an email or a phone call). When we got home from work there was a recorded delivery letter waiting for us. We now know what a letter from our agency looks like. We collected it from our neighbour and ceremoniously opened it at the kitchen table. It was from the agency and stated '*you have been successful and approved as adopters*'. We hugged and I shed a little tear. We were getting ready to crack open a bottle of fizz and I thought I had better check my email for the final time today. There it was, sitting in my inbox, an email from our social worker with the subject '*Matching update*'. We nervously opened it. She informed us that within our agency there are currently 47 adopters in the system, and 16 of those are Fostering for Adoption approved. There are five Fostering for Adoption babies aged from five months to two years all of which have Placement Orders imminent and two Fostering for Adoption babies about to be born in June. Given the nature of Fostering for Adoption, we are not able to have access to their profiles.

This email was a reminder that the ball is completely out of our court; it is up to the social workers to choose us as potential adopters. I am feeling emotional about this if I am honest. On the one hand we have been approved for a baby, for Fostering for Adoption, but now we know the numbers of approved adopters and children in the system, it has made us question how we are going to know that the baby that comes along is going to be the right fit for us? How long are we going to have to wait? Nobody knows. I have thought all along that it would probably happen quite quickly, but today has reminded us that we are part of a complex system and a lot needs to be worked through before a child is placed with us.

23 May

Today I felt better. I had a lovely catch up with my 'adoption friend' (who we met on our first training day). We spoke about our anxieties, worries and hopes for the future. It is reassuring to hear that our feelings are not too dissimilar; we are fortunate to have found each other. I really think we just have to be patient. Our time will come. During the training we hadn't really considered the 'competitive element' of the process, but now we know that we are being considered alongside 16 other couples, some of whom are now our friends, this is tough. If we are a match for either of the little ones to be born in June, then so be it, that will be our time – if not, then it will be someone else's perfect match and best for them and the child. If this is the case we will just wait a little longer. We have to think rationally. This afternoon I went for a walk with a good friend, again she was so lovely and supportive. We talked about life's ups and downs and how sometimes things don't work out as expected. Throughout this whole process our close friends have been with us every step of the way, and we are so grateful.

26 May

We have just returned from three nights camping. Every year, ten or so families from our street go away together. I spent most of the time thinking that next year another little person will hopefully be joining in the annual camping trip. I just can't wait. We are so fortunate to have found this village; everyone is so friendly and it is a perfect place to bring up a child. I often think about the phrase *'it takes a village to raise a child'* and I am sure each and every one of our neighbourhood friends, those on our street and from the wider community, will have an important part in our little one's life. We have recently announced via email to our youth group that we will soon be adopting. We felt it was important for parents to be able to discuss this with their children. We didn't want the young people in the group wondering where a baby had suddenly appeared from. We have been so overwhelmed with lovely messages and emails. I also can't believe that several of the parents have come back to us and said that they themselves are adopted.

1 June

Some time ago we booked a paediatric first aid course, a requirement of our agency. The course was in my parents' hometown and run by St John's Ambulance. We went with my mum and dad. It was excellent and informative. Will and I used it as a refresher but this was the first time my parents had had any form of first aid training. It was a good day and we all came away feeling positive that we are now more knowledgeable.

9 June

My best friend has been today and has given us the most amazing gift. All of our friends have bought us a children's book that they love, what a thoughtful idea. It just makes me really happy to know that all of these people are going to be around to help us. It just shows what a lot of love people have to give and this is going to be one very loved child. With Fostering for Adoption I have always felt uneasy about having a baby shower. Part of me felt it wasn't appropriate yet another part of me felt like it was another loss, something else I was missing out on. My best friend knew that I wasn't keen on the idea, so she hatched the 'book plan' instead. We now have 45 children's books – a mini library to read to our little one.

12 June

We had a call from our social worker this afternoon. She said that our profile is one of two that has been put forward for the two babies to be born in June. We don't know anything else. There is a matching meeting tomorrow that she will attend so we will find out more then. I can't stop smiling. I really hope this isn't going to end in disappointment, but she sounded quite optimistic and I am not sure she would have told us if we weren't in with a chance.

14 June

I went to see my granny today. She is in a care home with dementia. I tried to have a conversation with her about adoption. It is so difficult, I am sure she doesn't know who I am. I told her about us being approved to adopt a baby, she said, *'That is exciting, a girl or a boy?'* *'I don't know'*, I replied. She said she has only ever had girls, which is true. That was the end of the conversation. It is a comfort to remember that pre-dementia she would have been delighted for us and would have welcomed a little one with open arms into her family. I told her that I loved her and we had a cuddle. This time she actually responded, *'I love you too'* – she hasn't said this in years. This really touched me, especially today, while we are waiting for news.

15 June

During our training we were asked if we wanted to be in a WhatsApp group with others on the course; at the time, we thought this was a brilliant idea, to be able to compare notes with our peers. However, during the matching phase this has become difficult. What we hadn't really thought about was that these seven families in our group are in the same pool of approved adopters; we are being considered for the same babies and children. This is hard. I am so relieved that the couple whom we are the closest to have different adoption requirements; we opted for one child, they are waiting for a sibling group.

Both of us had hoped that we would have been matched and placed by now, but we are still waiting. Today we met up with them in a pub halfway between our homes. We had a lovely meal and compared notes on social workers, the process, decorating baby rooms, our fears and excitement for what was to come. Let's hope that next time we meet, both of us will have had some good news to share.

17 June

I am feeling stressed. The social worker called to speak about a potential Fostering for Adoption placement. She went through the paperwork that needs to be completed and the logistics of how it happens. What I felt was missing was a more in-depth discussion about the decision that is made and how we are meant to know that this is the right baby for us. So many people say that you know when it is a perfect match, but how will we know?

I have not really felt like this before. I couldn't get it out of my head or distract myself. Will was away, so a friend came round for a chat. After talking through it, I was a little clearer on why I was feeling like this – I am struggling to manage the uncertainty with work. It feels like when you are finishing to go on holiday, that feeling of wanting to get the 'to-do' list done and wrap everything up. However, the problem with this process is that you don't know when 'the holiday' is going to begin and you will be off work for a year. This is really tricky.

18 June

This afternoon we had a lovely time sorting through the baby clothes, the muslins, the nappies, the sling and all the other things we might need. I can't quite believe it. We have waited years to do this and now we are packing a baby bag and deciding which outfit is going to be the first one he or she wears. Will has been sorting out the milk formula machine and we are probably going to fit the car seat soon. So, we are ready, just in case one of these babies is meant to be.

24 June

The tables turned again today. This afternoon we had a call about another baby that has just been born. Our social worker gave us a brief overview of the child's circumstances and the scenario which has led to the decision for it to be placed under Fostering for Adoption. When the call came through I was working at home. I grabbed the all-important 'adoption notebook' and scribbled everything down. This was a concealed pregnancy (hence wasn't on the radar of the agency) and the birth mother had previous children removed from her care. She had a history of concealing pregnancies and then abandoning the babies in the hospital post-birth. This is what had happened at the weekend. The baby was born, withdrawing from heroin, and is currently waiting to be discharged on a Fostering for Adoption placement once the medical team are happy that it is strong enough to leave. The baby is on its own, birth father is unknown. Our social worker has given us until tomorrow morning to make a decision. We need to decide if we want to meet the child's social worker and potentially go ahead with this placement.

We have spent hours talking about this baby; we have also spoken to our parents. Will's mother has expertise as a retired nurse and we asked her to do some research for us on babies who are withdrawing from drugs, specifically heroin. Yes, during our training we had done some research about drug withdrawal in babies, but it is not until you are presented with a case, where you need to make a quick decision, that you really need all the research that you can get. We have read that babies are tested within hours of birth against 16 criteria. Drug withdrawal most commonly shows between 24 and 72 hours and depends on 'the most recent history of drug dose and half-life of that drug ... short-acting substances like Heroin withdrawal can be seen within the first 24 hours ... long-acting agents like Methadone ... 1–3 days after birth' (Shukla et al, 2020). Signs of withdrawal include tremors, high pitched crying, irritability, length of sleep after feeding, hyperactivity, increased muscle tone, seizure, temperature, sweating, low heart rate and sickness (Shukla et al, 2020). This is anxiety-inducing reading material for any potential parent making a life-changing decision. If a baby was withdrawing, they would be monitored and given a sedative or morphine to wean off the drug. We also read that withdrawing babies can be hard to settle and to comfort, in which case, skin to skin contact is important. The long-term impact of neonatal drug abuse is unknown, which means that adopters are taking huge risks accepting babies who are born withdrawing. Fortunately we have been able to get access to medical journals; without this information we would have felt very much in the dark.

We spent a few hours talking and finally came to a decision. In the morning we will let them know that we don't think this is the right match for us – taking on a withdrawing baby is just too much for us. We are so sad. There is a tiny baby lying in hospital with nobody to care for it. We really hope that there is someone out there, and for them this will be the baby they are waiting for. We are exhausted, what a decision to have to make.

25 June

Today I was the lead organiser for a big event at work – it was an important day. I tried to call our social worker at 9am but there was no answer. I had to leave one of my meetings at 10am, to call her quickly from the corridor. Will and I had chatted again this morning before we left for work; for us, last night we had made the right decision. I felt like I needed to speak to our social worker as soon as possible so they could start to make contact with other potential adopters. I was still sad to think of the baby all on its own in hospital – although I know that of course it was receiving wonderful care by hospital staff. I felt like we had abandoned the baby, just as its birth mother had done. It is so hard to think rationally when you are so emotional. I managed to have a quick chat with our social worker; she understood the decision we had come to and acknowledged that it must have been hard for us. The event at work was a success, and I was quite relieved to have a distraction. We have made the right decision for us. We have to keep believing in the system, and no, we will never know the outcome for this baby, but hope that the right match is found.

During our training and assessment we were repeatedly told about the potential risk of drug abuse on unborn babies and to be prepared for withdrawal from cocktails of harmful substances. It was not until our experiences during matching that the impact of this really hit us. Will the baby be in intensive care? What will be the immediate impacts? What are the likely long-term impacts? So many unknowns. Here Hannah and Claire share their experience of accepting a baby withdrawing from drugs: the immediate challenges, longer-term impacts and uncertainties.

Our first daughter's birth mother was a prolific drug user. Before we accepted the placement we did lots of research. We watched videos on YouTube of withdrawing babies and listened to the piercing cries they make – we were not put off. The birth mother stopped drinking once she knew she was pregnant, so the risk of foetal alcohol syndrome (FAS) was minimal, but she was addicted to a large number of drugs and continued to take these throughout her pregnancy. Our daughter was born at 37 weeks but only weighed 4lbs; she was undernourished and hadn't had the chance to thrive. She was born tremoring which continued for many months after birth. The signs of withdrawal were not instant, it took four days before she started showing symptoms. Birth mother admitted to using four bags of heroin while in labour so we knew the side effects would come. All babies respond differently to neonatal abstinence syndrome. Our first daughter was given morphine and weaned off it over ten days in hospital relatively easily. Our second daughter was readmitted to hospital at three months old for further morphine as she was struggling so much. Both birth mothers had similar drug habits. From our research we were aware that most children born withdrawing have behavioural issues, longer term – this is the greatest evidenced response to in utero drug exposure. What we weren't aware of was some of the other issues that we may face. Both of our girls have horrific gastro problems and as babies they had multiple allergies, likely caused by underdeveloped bowels. Our eldest also had issues with her limbs, she could barely bend until she was well over one – her muscles where so tight from the early withdrawals.

Our eldest is the sweetest, kindest and funniest child you could meet – she is loved by everyone who meets her. She is her. A tiny little crazy human who had to battle so much so early on and has come out the smartest little fighter. Will we face issues in the future? Almost certainly. Impulse control and sensory processing are already showing to be challenging – but would we change her, never. Our youngest is still struggling at nearly a year old but she was also exposed to large amounts of alcohol.

No two children are the same regardless of their early life experiences and it's so precious to watch them both grow. The most important part of our role as parents is to be their biggest advocates. We know when what they are doing is normal and when something isn't right. We have been and will be working hard to get them the help they need and deserve.

(Hannah and Claire, Foster to Adopt/Fostering for Adoption, girl, one week old)

7 July

We have had a quiet week on the adoption front. I am relieved. After the decision we had to make, I think we needed some time to reflect and move on. To some extent, it has helped us as we now know what to expect next time. We now know that the call can come at any time. We get brief details, we are expected to make a quick, often overnight decision, we need to do some more research on drug withdrawal, and importantly, we know that it is possible to be offered a newborn baby.

Today it was my sister-in-law's baby shower. I am sure that most people who are reading this book will know how hard these events are for those who have struggled with fertility and miscarriage, indeed anyone who is childless, not out of choice. I can now add to this list, those being in the 'waiting' phase for an Adoption Placement. In recognising the potential angst that I may be experiencing, my wonderful mother-in-law had prepared a baby gift bag for both of us. She gave me mine before leaving for the baby shower – an acknowledgement that we have a baby coming too, we just don't know who or when.

8 July

I woke up this morning feeling extremely nervous, the sort of nerves you get when you are about to sit an exam or something really important is about to happen. We had stayed at my in-laws so I drove into work from their house. As I passed through the city my attention was drawn to a banner that said the words 'Foster' and 'Adopt'. I just had a feeling that today we were going to get a call from our social worker.

I was busy all day but kept checking my email in anticipation. It was 4:15pm, I was driving home, sitting in traffic and I got a call. My phone flashed 'social worker'. I immediately pulled over to speak to her, notebook at the ready. She was ringing with information about another baby that we had been selected for. I really can't believe that this might be happening. The baby will be born by C-section on Thursday. It sounds like the social workers want us to make a decision on Wednesday, before the baby has been born. This sounds like a massive ask, so we are not really sure what is going to happen. How can we make a life-changing decision before the baby has been born? So far we have been given scant details of the background of the birth mother; however, despite the fact we know less about this baby than the previous one, we just feel a connection to it, something we can't quite put a finger on. We have a feeling that this baby is meant for us.

Sitting in the layby, I said to our social worker that I needed to speak to Will before making a decision about a potential meeting on Wednesday. Will is on his way back from a business trip abroad. I rang him, me in a layby, him at an airport about to board a plane – trying to have a life-changing conversation. It was a 'yes' we are interested and would like to meet with the social worker to find out more about the baby and its background – for us to be able to make an informed decision. Before getting on the motorway, I stopped at a supermarket, I thought I had best stock up on newborn nappies, just in case a baby was going to be making an appearance this week. When I got home I spoke to our parents and then later on in the evening managed to speak to Will again while he was in a taxi on the way back from the airport.

It is now 10:30pm. Will will be home soon but we must get some sleep; we have got quite a week ahead of us. I have also had to make a decision given this news. At the end of the week, I am supposed to be in Cardiff at an event which I have co-organised. However, as we may be accepting a baby on Friday, there is no way I am going to be able to go. I have sent an email tonight to my colleagues and I will speak to them tomorrow.

I am really trying not to get too excited. This could be our baby that is going to be born this week, a baby that could be with us for the rest of our lives. As I have said before, if it is meant to be, it is meant to be.

10 July

We hardly slept last night, anxious and excited about our meeting this morning with the social workers. We were up early to give the house a quick clean before everyone arrived. Unlike our home visits we decided that the kitchen table was a better place for this kind of meeting – for note-taking and paperwork. Once the social workers arrived we did quick introductions and made drinks for everyone. It ended up being an intense four and a half hour meeting. The social worker started at the very beginning. He had been involved with the family for years and had been the lead social worker on the case; he was able to answer all of the questions we asked him. Of course I can't share the full account and details of what we were told, but we were left shocked by the scenario which was laid out in front of us. This was the case of a young mother who had the world turned against her. At a very young age she ran away from home, she had been in and out of care herself; she was a victim of child sexual exploitation and domestic violence, as well as a prolific drug user. With the father(s) in prison, this was now her fourth baby, the previous three had all been taken into care. The other children have all experienced abuse and neglect and have developmental delay likely caused by drug and alcohol abuse during pregnancy. This, her fourth pregnancy, was concealed – up until last week social services didn't know she was pregnant. We were told that once a birth parent with a history of child removal attends any medical facility the system is triggered. In this case, the birth mother had been in pain and last week attended Accident and Emergency. The scan revealed that she was near term, so they booked her in for a C-section on Thursday as she had complications with previous pregnancies. The gender of the baby is unknown.

On Monday, a team of professionals met to discuss the unborn baby, and it was agreed that a plan of Fostering for Adoption should be put in place. The reported father (a DNA test would be done after the birth) is well known to the police with a string of criminal convictions and while a parenting assessment would need to take place, we were told that it is highly unlikely that the baby would be able to be placed with him.

By the end of the four and a half hours we were emotionally drained. I have to say we didn't feel at all pressured to say that we would accept the baby, unlike how this had been communicated to us at the beginning of the week. At the end of the meeting Will and I were both of the opinion that we should wait and make a decision once the baby was born. Our main concern was the impact of drug abuse. Post-birth we would be called and told the baby's initial vitals and on that basis we would make a decision. We spent the rest of the afternoon doing as much research as we could on the names of drugs that we knew the birth mother had been taking.

One of the hardest aspects about this process is the confidential nature of the information we are being told. Here I have written scant details; the depth of the trauma and abuse that we are making our decision on is extreme. We have been told not to discuss these details with anyone and this is what we find really difficult. We speak to our parents about all major life decisions and this feels completely unnatural not to discuss it with them. We did call them after the meeting and gave them a brief outline of the scenario and aired our initial thoughts.

This afternoon I had to go for a walk to try and process the situation we were in. I decided to go and have a quiet five minutes sitting in our local church. As I sat there, I made a request *'if this is the right baby for us, please give me a sign.'* A little while later I left the church, closed the door behind me and walked down the pathway. Then, out of nowhere came the most ear-piercing alarm. It stopped me in my tracks and I soon realised it was coming from the church. I was mortified; I couldn't believe I had accidentally set off the church alarm. My second thought – *'what kind of a sign is that? A warning sign?'* Fortunately, in a panic I managed to contact someone with access to the alarm code. What a drama.

We are going to bed tonight thinking that tomorrow we could be parents to this newborn baby. I feel completely drained. We made the decision that if the baby is initially showing positive signs then we will accept and take the risk of the longer-term unknowns. We are going to sleep wishing the baby lots of love as it makes its arrival into the world tomorrow.

11 July

Oh goodness, what a day, I don't even know where to begin. I am so sad. I was working at home this morning and Will went into work. I was quite grateful that I had a report to be working on; it took my mind off what was about to happen. We didn't know what time to expect the call, so I had the phone by me from the early hours. Well, we got 'the call' at 11:30am from the child's social worker. A baby boy had been born at 11am. He was healthy, doing well, there were no concerns, an incubator was not needed and he was a good weight. He didn't yet have a name and no tests, other than the initial vitals, had been done. I was asked what I thought and I said I would need to speak to Will. I quickly rang and we made the decision, on the basis of these good initial signs, we would go ahead and accept him. I rang back the social worker, he told us to sit tight and he would let me know the plans for the afternoon and when we could come and see the baby.

A few weeks ago, once we had been approved by the panel, I panicked – how would we know when the baby offered was 'the one'. Well, this felt just right. We thought this was the baby that would be part of our family. I couldn't believe it, it was happening. I spent the next few hours in a bit of a spin, going through the hospital bag, making sure everything was ready and rang our close friends and family to tell them the news.

What happened next completely took us off guard. There was a massive U-turn late afternoon. The social worker called again at 4:30pm; it was not good news. He told us that a family member had come forward and offered to take the baby. They were contesting the adoption. This was a family member that had previously told social services that they did not have the capacity to take care of the baby under a Special Guardianship Order. In the meeting yesterday the social worker had said that all avenues with family members had previously been explored and a baby coming to us on a Fostering for Adoption placement was 'last resort'.

The family member in question had visited the hospital this afternoon and they had changed their mind, they couldn't let the baby go. This is the end of the road for us. You can't make this up; it is unbelievable, we are so disappointed and sad. However, we have to hope that the best pathway for this baby is to stay with its extended family. I have cried so much this evening that I don't have any tears left in me.

12 July

I woke up with a throbbing headache; there are no words to describe how I feel. This week we have really been through the mill. The emotional energy we put into making this huge decision, only to be let down soon after, is the most draining thing we have ever experienced. Later on this afternoon we had another call from the baby's social worker. On the one hand I was surprised to hear from him, in fact him calling gave me a little hope that the tables may have turned again. We were told the name of the baby and that he had scored 9, twice, on the Apgar score (an initial test to indicate the health of a newborn baby). The top score is 10, so a 9 is very good. It seems that 24 hours post-birth he is doing really well. We were also told that the birth mother had already self-discharged and left the baby, which matched her history. The family member who came forward is now going to be assessed by social services. He did however leave the conversation open, in that he may come back to us if the assessment is negative. We don't really know how we feel about this – we may or may not hear about this baby again.

On Monday we had the initial call, on Wednesday a four and a half hour meeting, the baby born on Thursday, accepted the baby at lunchtime and were turned down by late afternoon. This is one of the raw edges of Fostering for Adoption. We are left feeling emotionally drained and so sad for the children in the system. Will and I have talked about this at length; we feel that we are well-educated, well-read, we watch the news and given our jobs we feel that we have a reasonable sense of what is going on in society and around us – but from what we have heard and experienced this week, we have no idea. It is so sad for the family and the children involved. We will never fully know his birth mother's circumstances, and the series of events that led her to walk out of hospital without him, but it reminded me about one of the activities that we did on one of our training days. We were told that families who adopt children from scenarios like the one described often have an urge to take the mothers under their wing as well – to help them get their lives on track and break the cycle of drug misuse, abuse and the devastation that goes hand in hand with this.

We are glad to see the back of this week.

15 July

I am away for a few nights to attend a work event I have spent a year co-organising. After last week I am now grateful for the distraction. It has been so lovely to get away, concentrate on work, eat nice food and meet new colleagues. Yes, my phone hasn't left my side in case we get another call, but the event is certainly helping to calm the nerves.

During our training and preparation for Fostering for Adoption, what had not been conveyed to us was the potential rollercoaster of matches, decision making and let-downs that adopters may experience. The overarching narrative that we were told was that 'it could be quick'. Yes, for some adopters of course it is quick with matching for some happening pre-panel but others wait over a year. In the case study below, Nellie and Louis speak of their wait for a Fostering for Adoption placement and the multiple matches and disappointments which followed. Yes, it can be quick once everything is in place, but the waiting can be agonising.

> It was a Wednesday morning, nearly a year after we had been approved to adopt – we had a phone call about baby Jess – 'a baby is due in a month, we don't know much about this pregnancy but we do have some information on birth siblings – can you meet on Friday with other social workers?' – YES, YES, YES.
>
> I was on my way home for the scheduled meeting with the social workers when I had another call – 'the baby has come early, she was born this morning, birth family have put a family member forward and the social worker is in court as we speak'. This was yet another blow to our Fostering for Adoption journey, baby number 6, each one went no further for one reason or another. Like the other five babies, we pushed Jess to the back of our minds, put on brave faces and waited for the next. Always excited but then came the disappointment and tears.
>
> Three months later the phone rang again, 'Do you remember the baby ... can you meet tomorrow?' – absolutely we can. This was the first time we had been told her name, it made her real – please let her be the one, it must be, she's come back, but let's not get our hopes up, it might not happen, it won't happen.
>
> The next day we met with the social workers. There wasn't much information about Jess as her birth mother hadn't engaged with services although there was slightly more information about her siblings. It was a quick meeting, we chatted, saw photos of her and cried – they said they would love her to be placed with us. Then came the three-week wait – waiting for paperwork, social workers on annual leave and ADM approval. She came home soon after – she was amazing. We did

have that niggle of worry about her returning to her birth family but we knew we could never hold back from giving her 100 per cent. We would give her our all whatever the final result, either staying with us as our daughter or if the unimaginable happened, she would take that love, care and attention with her as a base of confidence and self-esteem for her future.

(Nellie and Louis, Early Permanence Placement, girl, three months)

As you have read, we had the experience of a family member coming forward on the day of placement. Of course, this is the best scenario. However hard it was for us at the time there is no doubt that if we had been placed and then family members came forward, the uncertainty and risk would have been unbearable. For Elaine and James, this happened with both of their Fostering for Adoption placements: family members came forward and requested to be considered as permanent carers. This is their story.

During both placements we have had the experience of family members being proposed as permanent carers for our little ones. During our first placement a family member came forward, and then again during the court hearing for the Freeing Order (see the Adoption (Northern Ireland) Order (1987) for an explanation). This delayed the process and was worrying. During our second placement a family link became apparent just before the court hearing; this had to be followed up and investigated. We were told not to worry each time, but even when a lot of facts are known, you still have an anxious wait for a decision to be made.

This is an emotionally difficult route to adoption, to stand in the gap for as long as we are needed, to protect a child, while an organisation decides their future. It protects a child from moving from placement to placement, home to home. It protects them from the damage caused by multiple moves, it enables them to attach securely to a carer(s) and it enables their brain to grow and function normally without disruption or damage. Fostering for Adoption can seem hard but we would do it over and over knowing we take the brunt of it instead of a little one.

(Elaine and James, Concurrent Placement from birth,
a sibling to their three year-old)

19 July

We are now getting ready for our annual summer camp; we are taking 20 young people away for the best part of a week. This year, as you would expect, our plans have been complicated with the uncertainty surrounding the potential arrival of a baby. We planned for various scenarios in case both of us, or one of us, couldn't be on camp this year. All of our co-leaders and parents have been amazing, willing to step in and lend a hand if needed. We decided to make this camp local, so if we do need to leave if we 'get a call' then we can do.

26 July

Camp is always good for leaving your worries behind you, getting stuck in and having fun. When looking after 20 of other people's children, you don't really have a moment to think about yourself. In the assessment process, one of the negative points about us as a couple was that we didn't have any experience of children staying overnight at our house. We pushed back on this and made the case that taking 20 children away for a week trumps this – including hospital visits for injuries, dealing with illness in the middle of the night, friendship dramas and everything in between.

We are now back from camp and we have had an email from our social worker to say she hasn't heard anything about babies in the pipeline. Given this, we have made the decision that we need to go away on holiday for a week. We have booked a last-minute holiday to Greece for some sunshine, I can't wait. Now we have just got to hope we don't get a call while we are away.

1 August

We were up early to head to the airport. On the way, I had one final look at the portal before we switch off for the week. A new profile has been uploaded, three-year-old twin boys. My heart skipped a beat; they were gorgeous and instantly loveable. Currently in a foster home and awaiting a match. I showed Will their profile, he smiled and his instant response was *'there is no way we could do that'*. Something inside me is excited, I want to know more. We walked around the airport looking at all of the toddlers and imagining how we would cope with two; we saw a few twins and each time looked at each other and grinned.

By this stage in the matching process, I was starting to lose hope. My attachment to the twin boys on the portal was a coping mechanism. I needed to keep believing that this could happen, that we were going to end up with a child. For me, the twins on the portal were a potential answer. Yes, we would need to forego how we had imagined having a child would be, but here were two beautiful, blonde, blue-eyed, smiling children that needed a home. Despite this, I knew that they were not for us – I just needed to imagine what it might be like to get me through this stage. We needed to stick to what we had said from Day 1; deep down we wanted a baby. We wanted what Joanne and John describe below, to be able to provide a home to a newborn baby – to be part of their story from the very beginning.

> We were chosen for a Fostering for Adoption placement two weeks before he arrived and Adoption Leave started a few days before. We knew very little about him before he was born. Practically, we were ready, our generous friends had passed on all the essentials. Emotionally, we felt less ready – but I suppose all new parents feel like this. We knew the planned date for the induction and had been told to head to the hospital at 9:30am the following morning. That morning came and we still hadn't heard from our social worker. With no news, we made the decision to head to the hospital. We got the call on the way – our little boy had been born (up until that point we didn't know the sex of the baby) and he was a tiny 4lb 12oz.
>
> When we arrived at the hospital we were treated with such care by the staff on the maternity ward. They filled us in on the birth and birth mother's progress. We were able to feed our boy and change him into clothes that we had brought with us (they were far too big for him). We then waited to be discharged. The journey home was a blur, later my husband said he had never driven so carefully in his life. The next few days were full of midwives, social workers and health visitors – we felt incredibly well supported by all the professionals involved as we made the transition to looking after a newborn. It was such a

privilege that we were able to have so many firsts with our boy – first car journey, first bath and even first nappy explosion.

We spent the next three weeks all together, taking it slow, holding him, feeding him, going on walks and soaking up every moment. We took so many photos and journaled every detail so we would have physical memories to give him in the future.

(Joanne and John, Concurrent/Fostering for Adoption, boy, one day old)

Katie and Jack were also able to bring their baby home from hospital. In their case study below, they describe the flexibility needed on the part of adopters, being able to change plans last minute when babies arrive early and adapting to the shifting arrangements made by the team of professionals. They speak about the intense emotional pressure that new adopters face when they are responsible for a child in their care.

We were approved at panel in early May for Fostering for Adoption, we had everything ready. After many years of failed fertility treatment we were finally excited – the nursery was decorated and our friends and family were buying clothes and other bits for a baby. We were shown a profile and had a linking meeting in mid-July, the baby was due early August. Enough time to prepare, or so we thought. The very next day, after the linking meeting, little one was born.

We had always hoped that we would be able to visit a little one in hospital but we knew that it doesn't always happen. The initial plan was that three days after birth (due to birth mother's background) little one would be brought home to us by a social worker. This really scared me – meeting our little one for the very first time at our front door. Plans soon changed and we were fortunate that we were able to meet him for the first time in hospital. We stayed for hours – fed him, bathed him, had skin on skin, and above all, fell in love. The very next day, and only 48 hours after his birth, we were allowed to bring him home.

Having this experience and being with him from the very beginning was incredible. That was it, us and little one. No antenatal classes, no NCT groups, just us with a newborn who relied on us for everything.

He arrived during the global pandemic lockdown so our family weren't able to visit. We were by ourselves and had to learn quickly. After wanting a baby so desperately, for so long, the pressure to not get anything wrong was intense; we had to trust our instincts – we had to remember that we knew this little bundle better than anyone.

(Katie and Jack, Foster to Adopt, boy, two days old)

3 August

Over the past few days, we have talked a lot about the twin boys and have come to the decision that this was not what we have been preparing ourselves for. To be honest, I can't quite believe how attached to their profile I have become, as they are aged three, boys and there are two of them. We will keep riding this wave of uncertainty and see what is waiting for us around the corner.

I thought being on holiday would be a good break from everything; however, what has in fact happened is that we have had more time to think and talk. I am really going to try and perk up; I will bury my head in a few good books and try to focus on the positives rather than the unknowns.

I will never forget this holiday. The waiting and emotional toil were exhausting, we couldn't imagine what our life was going to be like because we had nothing to work with – we didn't know how this was going to end. It was hard. At the time of writing, Sarah and Alex are in a similar position. Below they describe how they are feeling as they wait for their match:

> We were led to believe that we would be matched with a baby the day after panel; we may have been naive but that is what we were told. They were keen to know if we had any holidays planned as during these dates we wouldn't be able to accept a baby; they wanted us to cancel any trips that we had already booked. We are now five months on and we don't have a child. It has been so difficult to manage with work. As the weeks and months have slipped by my colleagues must be really by wondering what on earth is going on. We are positive people, but this process is really testing us. This is our life and we are living it on a knife edge.
>
> (Sarah and Alex, Foster to Adopt, matching phase)

7 August

We are now back from our holiday. Apart from my meltdown at the beginning, we managed to switch off, relax, eat some lovely food, go on walks, swim and read our books in the sunshine. It was perfect and just what we needed to recharge our batteries. We are hoping to hear some news in the next few days, or at least an update on any potential children coming into the system.

21 August

We have had another call, another baby. We are referring to this one as number 7. After the third or fourth we felt we needed to number the children we have heard about or been offered. It was all getting quite confusing when speaking with each other and our close friends. As always, the social worker rang me. She sounded chirpy and a little excited. She had been contacted by a social worker who was interested in our PAR. She opened the conversation with '*boy, aged eight months*'. His Placement Order has already been granted and they are looking to place for straight adoption, rather than Fostering for Adoption. He has been in foster care since being discharged from hospital at birth and five other siblings have previously been adopted. All other children have developmental delay and the primary reason for removal was chronic neglect and domestic violence. Our social worker has been told that he is happy, smiling, babbling, easily comforted and currently meeting his developmental milestones. She then went on to explain that this case is much more straightforward and secure, unlike those on Fostering for Adoption placements which we have been considering. However, we would have to wait, this would not be an immediate placement. We would need to wait for the court hearing, our Matching Panel, introductions, transition and then he would move into our home. It would be highly likely that he would have already had his first birthday before moving in. I thanked our social worker for passing on the details and said that I would get back to her after speaking with Will. If I am honest, I knew from her opening sentence that this little one was not for us. For us, eight months is too old; if not a newborn then we will only really accept a baby under six months, as long as they are on a Fostering for Adoption placement. For us, we want the opportunity to build secure attachments at a young age. Soon after, we crafted an email to the social worker, explaining our decision. I also can't believe we have been offered *another* boy. We were told in the early days that we shouldn't have a preference, but deep down we have always imagined having a girl. Something is telling me that we are destined to have a boy.

We are both getting worried that the social workers might think we are being too fussy – how many can you be offered or be told about before you are put on some sort of blacklist? I have to say though, we are going to bed tonight calmer than we have been with the others. Once we had made the relatively quick decision we moved on – baby number 7 wasn't right for us.

22 August

This evening we started to crack on with another job that needed doing while we are waiting. We had previously decided not to do it as we wouldn't want a 'call' mid-job. We are sorting out the hallway, re-mortaring the brick flooring, painting the walls and building some shoe storage, for all those little shoes that will hopefully be passing through our hallway. It shouldn't take too long to do and will look good once it is finished. I can't believe we had the panic about finishing the kitchen and getting it ready in time for the panel. That was back in May, it is now August and we are still waiting.

Carrying on with life while waiting for a match is one of the hardest parts of this process. From booking holidays to completing jobs at home, you are in limbo. I remember someone comparing the 'waiting' phase of adoption to the third trimester of pregnancy. I would disagree. With pregnancy, there is the certainty that the baby will be born and there is a few weeks window of waiting. With the Fostering for Adoption process, you are approved at the panel and the baby can be placed at any time – days, weeks, months or even a year after the approval. This wait is complicated, fraught and emotional. In the case study below, Rachel describes her role as a nurse and how supportive her workplace were in facilitating a smooth transition to Adoption Leave, which happened at short notice:

> A few weeks after my Adoption Panel, I was contacted on Link Maker about a six-week-old baby boy. The following day there were several phone calls between my assessing social worker, the family finder and myself. I was told the baby's name, I'll call him Jack. Jack was currently in a parenting assessment placement with his birth mother but this had broken down. There was a court hearing that day which

concluded that Jack should be removed from the assessment unit and placed in a Fostering for Adoption placement. I was told there were three families being considered.

I was working full time as a nurse and contacted my manager to inform her that I was being considered for a Fostering for Adoption placement and if selected I would need to start my Adoption Leave very quickly. I explained that other families were also being considered and I thought it was unlikely that I would be chosen, being a single adopter. From the beginning I had been upfront about my adoption application and explained the Fostering for Adoption process to my workplace. My manager could not have been more supportive and agreed to rota my shifts after Adoption Panel in a way that would be easier to cover at short notice if I was to leave suddenly.

After several phone calls I heard at 4pm that I was the preferred prospective adopter and Jack would be placed with me ... the following day. I called my manager to explain what had happened and that I would need my year of Adoption Leave to begin with immediate effect. I was so lucky to have support from my workplace. She was very excited and completely fine about me leaving work so suddenly; this made the situation a lot easier to cope with.

(Rachel, Foster to Adopt, boy, six weeks)

1 September

The predicted weather forecast for the weekend was superb, so we decided to take advantage of it and book a last-minute canoe trip down the River Severn. It was amazing and I can't imagine that we will be doing anything like this for a while. We did six hours of canoeing per day and wild camped, magical. Perhaps *this* will be our last holiday before being placed, who knows?

We are now home. I am sitting in the nursery taking it all in, the mobile hanging above the cot, the drawers full of beautiful clothes, the toys in the basket, the prints hanging on the walls. The room is ready for a little human being that we don't know yet, but in an odd sort of way it is comforting to sit here.

From reading our account of the matching phase, the word rollercoaster springs to mind. In a moment our hopes are raised, only to be let down soon after. Sarah and Alex know this feeling of quick decisions and false hopes all too well. Below they describe a situation where they 'got the call' about a tiny baby not long after their Adoption Panel. Was this the one? Their baby?

> Three weeks after we had been approved we had a call from the family finder. She went through the details, it was a relinquished baby, six weeks old. We were told the ins and outs, what milk he was on, how much he drank, how much he weighed, the lot; I had two pages of notes about him. She asked us to have a think. Within 30 minutes of putting down the phone she rang back, *'he lives too close to you – it is too much of a risk that you would run into birth family'.* She said, *'well we need to stop this here because you won't have got attached'.* Unbelievable, this should have been looked at before they contacted us, our hopes and expectations had been raised.
> (Sarah and Alex, Foster to Adopt, matching phase)

7 September

Today we had the final adoption training course – we were due to do this back in May but we were unable to attend the specified date. The focus was 'Introductions and Transition'. The training wasn't compulsory but recommended. I have to say I was a bit sceptical about going, given that we were 90 per cent certain that we wanted to do Fostering for Adoption. Most of the content was aimed at toddlers and above, doing bump-ins in local parks (where the adoptive parents 'bump-in' to the child and carer in a public setting, often a park – the child at this stage won't know that this is their potential adoptive family), introductions followed by the transition. I think it would have been more beneficial to run a session specifically on Fostering for Adoption – the logistics and eventualities.

The most useful aspect was meeting other people, it was nice to chat with some of the other potential adopters. There was a real mix of people, some were in the early days of Stage 2 in the assessment process, others had just been approved, then there were those who had been waiting for months and one lady who had a match and was waiting for her Matching Panel.

The takeaway messages for us were *'be prepared'* and *'look after yourself'* during the transition process. I am going to use the rest of the time we are 'waiting' to make meals and stock up the freezer.

8 September

Another week has gone by, another week with no news. I still have the three-year-old twin boys on my mind; their profile is still on the portal. I think about them every day. Will said to me tonight *'Alice, I really think you need to stop talking about the twins.'* He is right, we need to move on and focus on what we have wanted from day one of this process, a baby.

CHAPTER 5

THE STORY CONTINUES: BEING MATCHED

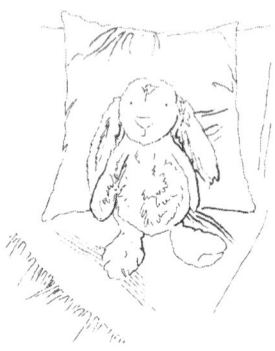

The intensity of the waiting phase is extreme. The cases and the system are complicated. It might seem arbitrary to number the children, but this was our way of keeping track. It was our way of remembering the babies we were told about, those we had seen profiles of, those that we were considered for and those we were offered. So, for all sorts of reasons, this led to us now being in September, five months on from the panel.

In this chapter we 'get the call'. This is about number 8, our number 8.

9 September

Today I was in London for an important presentation. My colleague and I had been invited to present at a conference. I left home in the morning and travelled by train. As I was going over my notes, I had another feeling. Was our social worker going to call? Was today going to be the day?

I made my way to a restaurant; my plan was to have lunch while going over my notes one last time. After ordering some food I got a message from our social worker; she asked if I was free and if I could speak. *Panic.* By this time it was 1pm and she said she was going to be in a meeting until 1:45pm. It was a long 45 minutes, my heart was racing. Of course, my plans to run through my presentation went out of the window. Just before 2pm, my notebook was out and I was ready for whatever news we were going to be told. Similar to the other 'calls' we had previously had, she went through the initial details of the case. This was a four-month-old baby boy (another boy) and she told me his name (my initial thought was *'that is a lovely name'*). She said he was a beautiful and happy baby. She went through the scenario that had led to him potentially being adopted. From birth he had been with a foster family and the social workers were hoping that the court would decide on Fostering for Adoption for placement. My gut feeling was this could be the one, this could be our little boy. My only reservation was that he was already four months old. I once again asked if she could give me half an hour to get hold of Will and talk it through with him. We were both positive and asked for a meeting with the allocated social worker.

Our social worker was pleased that we wanted to hear more. She reminded us that as we are now progressing with this baby, she would put on hold any other interest in our PAR. The time was now 3pm, I was due to meet my colleague so that we could have a final run-through of our presentation. I gave him brief details of what had just happened and we then focused on our notes and preparation. I couldn't quite believe the timing, I was about to give a critical presentation and we could have just heard the most important news of our adult life, news of a baby, our baby. Only time will tell how this pans out, but for now I am buzzing.

10 September

My phone rang at 9:20am this morning. Our social worker rang with news of a meeting on 17 September, at our house with both social workers. We are cautiously excited, we really hope everything works out this time.

11 September

Tonight Will and I managed to have a proper debrief about our latest news. We have been so busy since we had 'the call' and most of our conversations have been on the phone rather than face-to-face. We had a lovely dinner together and then began to write a list of everything we know about this baby – we feel really happy and have a good feeling that this is the baby for us.

14 September

We went shopping and allowed ourselves to buy something for him, obviously keeping the receipts, just in case. We bought him a lovely sleeping bag. This afternoon we sat down and wrote some notes ahead of our meeting with the social workers. On the basis of the information we have been told, we decided to write a list of positives and negatives about the case presented to us. After a good chat, we came up with a list of 18 positive points. These included: he is in good health, it seems that all avenues for maternal and paternal family members taking care of him have already been explored, he has brown hair like us, he has been well looked after and loved by the foster family from day one and, given the circumstances, placement needs to be as soon as possible. There are other positives that I can't write about due to confidentiality. In terms of negatives we could only think of two, one that we can't mention here but the other was that he was already four months old. My dream of a newborn placement would be over with this match. While we were very happy and excited, I couldn't get his age out of my head; in fact, I was upset, perhaps a newborn placement wasn't meant to be. We talked about this a lot and turned this negative into a positive. This four-month-old baby has been with a loving foster family from day one; he has had four months of secure attachments. Surely, this is much more important than my desire for a newborn?

To help us think this through, we then wrote a list of the positives and negatives of him being four months. There were 11 positives, including we know he is healthy and has had a good medical report; he will be more interactive than a newborn; he will still be a 'baby' needing milk and sleep; he will still be able to sleep in our room; we will still be able to carry him in a sling; and he should be in some sort of routine. In terms of the negatives there were two, first that we won't have known him from day one and secondly that for us it feels like another loss. Both of our lists had mostly positives. We couldn't help but be excited about this little one.

We then drew up a list of questions for the social worker. These included wanting to know about his birth mother and father, and the factors which have led to adoption, reasons why the wider family have been ruled out and how certain the social workers are that nobody is going to come forward at the last minute? What the likelihood is of contact sessions with birth parents, their frequency and location? Why the route of Fostering for Adoption has been chosen? What are the plans for post-adoption contact? What are the birth parents' feelings about the adoption, how likely are they to contest? What antenatal care did the birth mother receive and what are the results of any medicals that have been done? We also had lots of questions about the process, timings and the plan going forward. Of course we also had a list of questions which were specific to this baby; we wanted to know how much he weighed at birth, what time he was born, if he was born with hair, if it was a C-section or natural birth, how he has grown over the past few months and what are his routines and timings? So, so many questions about this little one that we can't wait to find out. The final question we have is *'why have we been chosen?'* This is something we really want to know, what drew the social worker to our profile? If this is the baby for us, we want this to be part of his story, knowing the reasons why our lives ended up converging.

I am now sitting on the floor in the nursery. This room has been ready since May. I often come in here, I find it a calm place to be. If I am talking to a friend on the phone or want time to think, I find myself sitting here. I am surrounded by clothes, books and teddies; it is a lovely room, ready for a little person. I have just spent the past hour sorting through the clothes that we have bought and been given. Given the news we have had this week, it looks like we will be needing the next size, 3–6 months from our friends. Giving back the newborn and 0–3 months clothes is hard, but I need to move on and start to get excited.

We have been told that if we accept this baby, this little boy could be with us next week. However, after our experiences over the summer, we have to be prepared that this isn't going to work out. We want to get excited; this could be it, this could be our baby. This could be the little person that joins our family forever, we can't wait.

15 September

A group of friends and I occasionally meet for a 'craft-er-noon', where we each bring a craft project we are working on, have a chat, drink tea and eat cake.

I decided that it might be a good idea to make our Christmas cards – over four hours I printed over 80 cards. An imminent baby arrival has certainly pushed up productivity once again. Later in the afternoon our neighbour popped around and gave us all the 3–6 month boy's clothes that we would need, it is so kind of her. I have photographed it all so I remember who has lent us what; it's going to be hard to keep track.

For so long I tried to imagine what it would be like to meet our baby, what would happen? How would we feel? Would we collect the baby from hospital or perhaps meet via a foster carer? To be honest it is so hard to imagine when there are so many variables. This is one of the reasons why I decided to write this book, I wanted potential Fostering for Adoption carers to be able to imagine what it might be like to accept a baby on a Fostering for Adoption placement. In the case study below, Rachel tells us what it was like for her when she was placed with Jack – in this case, Rachel collected Jack from a parenting assessment unit.

> After updating work, family and friends about Jack's imminent arrival, my mother and I made a mad dash to the shops for some essentials. I hadn't bought much in advance, given that I didn't know the age or gender of the child I would be matched with. I had decorated a bedroom in neutral colours and bought a cot bed which could be used for a variety of ages as well as a few books. I was unsure what Jack would arrive with so I kept the receipts in case they weren't needed. Everything felt so surreal. The following morning I made up his 'next to me' style cot and a bouncy chair so he would have somewhere to sleep and play when he arrived. I kept everything else in its packaging, I was sure something was bound to go wrong.
>
> The social workers arrived and shared some more information about Jack and his birth family. They asked me some questions about how I would manage potential difficulties and uncertainty and then took a look around my home. There was a lot of paperwork being shared between the social workers. It all felt a little rushed and chaotic, I was just excited to meet Jack and trusted the social workers to sort all of the formalities. We then left my house to collect Jack. I drove with my social worker and we met Jack's social worker at the parenting assessment unit.

Jack's birth mother was no longer resident in the unit but there were other families there with their babies. We were shown into a living area where there was a baby being held and another baby in a bouncy chair. I was unsure which was Jack until we were introduced. Seeing him for the first time took my breath away. I remember thinking he was the most beautiful baby I had ever seen. I couldn't believe how tiny he was and how lucky I was to be chosen to care for him.

The staff had supported Jack and his birth mother since he was a few days old. They explained that he would need lots of stimulation as he was often sleepy; he fed 3–4 hourly and needed waking for feeds. Several staff members came to see him and there were some photographs taken of everyone together which are now part of Jack's life story book. I gave him a bottle while my social worker took his belongings out to the car. The drive home felt like forever; there was a lot of traffic and I just wanted to get him home, it was getting late. Jack took it all in his stride and slept for most of the journey. When we arrived home my social worker had to leave but my best friend was waiting for us. She had set up a baby gym and bought Jack some presents, it was so wonderful. This was the most intense and overwhelming day of my life (and Jack's).

(Rachel, Foster to Adopt, boy, six weeks)

Like Rachel, Kristie is a single adopter. In her case study she describes getting ready for the twins to arrive – after the formalities of matching, they were brought to her house by the social worker and foster carer.

In the lead up to the twins coming home the emotions were overwhelming, I was excited and nervous at the same time. I loved the feeling of having everything ready for their arrival, although it was a mad dash to prepare – it was two weeks from having said 'yes' to them arriving. I bought the pram within half an hour of my social worker calling. It was a big expense, particularly with Fostering for Adoption, but I wanted to do it and I needed to be positive that all was going to work out. I set up the Moses baskets by my bed, their nursery was ready, the bottles washed and sterilised – I was ready for them to arrive.

We were in Covid lockdown when they were placed. I live with my mother, so we both had to self-isolate for two weeks beforehand. This added a further complexity as we had to order everything online and keep our fingers crossed that they would arrive on time. The twins were living with a foster carer, so we had a few phone calls to check details and practicalities. On the day of placement, the foster carer brought the twins to our house. The family finder social worker was also there for the handover, but she stayed in the car and asked through the window if I was okay. Our other social worker came into the house; she went through the paperwork but didn't stay long.

(Kristie, Early Permanence Placement, twins aged six weeks)

17 September

Written in the morning before our social worker meeting

Last night we spent most of the evening cleaning the house; of course, we wanted to make a good impression to the child's social worker. I hardly slept, it is so hard not to get too excited. This could be 'our morning', the one where it all works out and we go ahead and accept this little baby. Will said to me when we woke up *'do you think today is going to be our time to become parents?'* Of course I really hope so, but I don't want us to be disappointed again. I think we need to take one day at a time. Our social worker is due at 9am. She suggested we meet half an hour before to check that we are both okay and to run through any questions we may have, then the child's social worker will be here at 9:30am. As this case is Fostering for Adoption, we are not allowed to see any of the formal paperwork, everything has to be verbal. In other cases we instantly had the impression that the social workers really knew the family and case well, rather than referring to notes or reading from someone else's case file. I hope this happens with this little baby. I have had some lovely messages from our friends this morning; everyone is thinking about us which is comforting. Let's see what the next few hours bring.

Written in the evening

What a day we have had. We are absolutely buzzing, we can't quite believe it. The meeting went brilliantly. First, we had a chat with our social worker, as ever she was cautious with her approach; it is clear that she doesn't want us to be ruled by our hearts and is always highlighting the risks with Fostering for Adoption and any uncertainties which surround the scenario of the baby. It is much better this way, because of course, the placement needs to be right for us, and right for the baby. When the child's social worker arrived she immediately put us at ease. Of course I can't share any of the specific details but she started by saying *'he is a four-month, beautiful, happy and settled baby'*, and said she had chosen us because we looked like him. At this point I wondered if all social workers tell prospective adopters that the babies are beautiful and they have similar features to potential parents. I was quite sceptical. She said that he loves interaction and has developed secure attachment with his foster carers.

She quickly got out her notes and started from the very beginning. She has been the allocated social worker from the early days of conception, working with the family for well over a year. Early on, the baby was put on the Child Protection Register, meaning that the birth mother would be monitored closely by social services as her pregnancy progressed. Throughout the pregnancy, interventions were put in place and the court ruled when the baby was born that she and the baby should be placed immediately in a mother and baby foster care placement. We were pleasantly surprised that these existed. We had heard about and seen on television mother and baby units, which had a very institutional feel, but we didn't realise that some placements also happened with families, in homes. The social worker was confident that she and the baby had received the best package of care. Unfortunately, however, a series of assessments and events led to the decision being taken by the team that the baby should be placed for adoption. All other family members had been considered and parenting assessments had come back negative, which meant that they were not deemed suitable by social services to take care of the baby.

From our experience, we were keen to know how certain the social worker was that the baby was going to be placed for adoption, and hopefully Fostering for Adoption. She explained that the baby's guardian is supportive of the plan for adoption and our understanding is that they hold quite a bit of weight in the process. This sounds positive. Going forward, the plan would be for no face-to-face contact with the birth family. The social worker stressed that she wanted this to be a Fostering for Adoption placement, to help support secure attachments from a young age. She was also relatively optimistic that the

Fostering for Adoption stage would be relatively short and we could move to the Matching Panel and an Adoptive Placement as soon as possible.

During the meeting, we were asked if we wanted to see a photograph of the baby. This was a tense moment, I wasn't prepared for this. I didn't think this would be an option. She had brought with her a photograph that the foster carers had taken. I was so nervous, I just didn't know what to expect; this could be our son we were looking at. I took one look and I was shocked. It was a photograph of his head and shoulders and right next to his head was the face of a dog. My first thought was, *'that dog shouldn't be that close to his face'* – in the 30 seconds or so that we were shown the photograph, I spent most of the time distracted by the dog. Sadly we couldn't keep the photograph. With Fostering for Adoption placements, no photographs or any identifying documents are allowed to be kept. Once the social workers had left one of the first things I asked Will was if he looked properly at the photograph. He reassured me that he wasn't distracted by the dog and the baby was beautiful.

Our three-hour meeting was so positive. It was obvious as the meeting progressed that this was clearly the baby for us. Will and I didn't really need to have a chat with each other before making the decision. We could just tell from reading each other that this was our baby. This was going to be the little boy that we were going to welcome into our lives.

We got such a good feeling from his social worker. We felt that she and her team want the best outcome for this little boy. Coming out of the meeting I really wanted to make sure I felt that adoption was the best decision for this baby, and I did. It really makes me sad that our happiness is a result of a terrible situation; however, we have to turn this around and look forward. If this placement is meant to be, we will love him unconditionally and one day he may be reading this.

The social workers have now left and I am sitting in his room. This is finally happening, I can't believe it.

In about 20 minutes we are going on camp – our last weekend as a family of two will be spent in a field looking after 27 children. We have been told we should hear more on Monday.

We made the call to our parents, to say how well the meeting had gone and that we were going ahead. This is one call they will vividly remember; they are riding this wave of uncertainty with us. My mum and dad were about to board a flight to go on holiday – they had been nervously waiting for our news.

Baby we are ready for you, more ready than you will ever know.

21 September

We have been told that we need to have a 'transition teddy' for our little one. They recommend that we sleep with the teddy for a few nights so that it picks up our smell. This morning we went into town and selected 'Bunny' – he is gorgeous, soft and cuddly.

We can't wait for Bunny to meet our little one. Tonight, he will join us in bed.

23 September

We had hoped that we would get a call today to say that the Fostering for Adoption placement was going ahead. However, it turns out that the professionals had planned for his case to be Fostering for Adoption but this had not yet been through court, so this is what we are waiting for. Hopefully once the judge has made the decision, he will move to us immediately on a Fostering for Adoption placement. I am in work today and I have primed everyone that this is imminent.

At 6pm we had a call from our social worker, it isn't great. It hasn't all fallen through, which obviously would be devastating, but the goal posts have been moved. The trouble is we don't understand the process and every case is different. It seems that things have changed since last week and now we have been told that we need to wait another week for various decisions to be made about the Fostering for Adoption placement. I am most sad to think he is another week older; I just want him here as soon as possible. He is now close to five months old, getting older by the day. This process is excruciating. I now need to explain this to my family, friends and colleagues. Another week to wait.

26 September

I have spent the last few days in what I can only describe as a thick fog. I am really tired and feeling drained. I have started doing some batch cooking; he will soon be weaning so at least we can be prepared.

30 September

Our social worker rang this morning, we are one step forward. We are now waiting for an emergency court hearing; this will be to make the final decision as to whether he can move to us on a Fostering for Adoption placement. It is sounding positive (everyone in his team wants this to happen, rather than the standard adoption route); we have been told if they can get into court today or tomorrow then introductions will start this week. This afternoon they are sending over the plan for introductions, a staggered process for us to integrate into his life. We are trying to not get too excited, who knows what's going to happen in court.

1 October

Another difficult work decision to make. At the end of this week I am co-organising an event, obviously I haven't booked a hotel yet. My colleagues are being very understanding, but I don't want to let them down if the baby isn't going to be placed this week. I have decided to make a last-minute decision on this and book the hotel on the day, if I am able to go.

3 October

This afternoon I spoke to our social worker; there has been *'no news from the guardian'*. We are getting mixed messages about what we are actually waiting for, it is so confusing. The guardian has verbally said to the social worker that in principle she agrees with a Fostering for Adoption placement. We have now been told that the paperwork is stuck with the legal team. I am so sad another week has gone by. I have booked my hotel for the event and I will leave at 4:30am tomorrow morning.

4 October

It was an early start but I made it to the event with an hour to spare. The morning sessions were a good distraction. During the afternoon while chairing a session, my phone, on silent, flashed 'social worker'. My heart skipped a beat. Obviously I couldn't answer but my mind was racing. I had to wait until the session had ended, then managed to escape and call her from the corridor. She was only calling to say there had been no news. So disappointing. I am going to bed tonight with Bunny, he has come with me for comfort – hopefully soon he will be snuggled in the cot with our little one.

7 October

We are fuming. We heard today that the guardian needs to sign the paperwork and make her recommendation to the court. This is what we were told two weeks ago. I really can't see the baby arriving this week. I am finding it so difficult with work – it appears that I am making it up. I asked if we could have a photograph of him, sadly because the court hasn't made the decision, we are not allowed to have any paperwork or photographs related to him. We only saw the one photograph of him (and the dog) for about 30 seconds; I can't really remember what he looks like. I just want to look at his little face.

10 October

We have had a difficult few days. Will's dad has been diagnosed with heart failure and is really poorly. With this and the conflicting information we are getting from the social workers we feel that we are living life on the edge. In one call we are told that it could happen any day, almost immediately, and then a day later we are told that if the court doesn't agree with the plan of Fostering for Adoption, we need to prepare ourselves that it could be months before he is placed. To add to our upset, our social worker has told us that she will be leaving and is going to work for another department in Children's Services. The person that we have spent a year building up a relationship with, the one who knows us inside out, the one who we have opened up our lives to and the one looking out for us is leaving. We are waiting to hear who our new social worker will be. We understand that people move on to new roles but this is really bad luck that it has happened to us, at this stage. It is so upsetting and unsettling. Another week goes by.

As I have written elsewhere in this book, one of the most frequently voiced risks and concerns with Fostering for Adoption is the potential of the baby being returned to the birth family. In the case study below, Hannah and Claire speak about the decisions which were made in the early days of their placement. This shows how quick the tables can turn and how risky the process is, from the very beginning:

> We had accepted an unborn baby on a Fostering for Adoption placement. Her birth family had all been assessed to care for her and there was no viable options for placement. This all happened relatively quickly and two weeks later she was born.
>
> We were due to meet her the day after she was born. However, it wasn't as smooth as we hoped. From the maternity ward she went straight to the Special Care Baby Unit; there were no major problems but she needed the extra support. Suddenly, post-birth the social workers were saying that *'we don't want you to get too attached if it all goes wrong.'* Attached? We were head over heels in love with her already. We had spent two weeks buying her tiny baby clothes, a cot, bottles and everything you normally would have nine months to prepare for. We weren't allowed see or hold her. Every day we rang our social worker and begged them to let us meet her.
>
> Finally, after a very long week, we were allowed to meet her. She was perfect. We visited every day for a week, leaving only a few hours each day to allow for birth family to visit. A week later I was at the hospital while my partner was at work, I had a feeling something had happened. The nurses seemed strange, like they were avoiding me. I overheard a phone call from one of the nurses *'what are we supposed to do with foster mum?'* she said. As I sat feeding our little girl an email came through. It was from our social worker to say that her birth grandad had not known about her and he now wants custody. Over the past week he had an assessment, it was positive – the children's team wanted me to leave the hospital and not return. Our little girl was to be discharged into conventional foster care while the care plan was sorted. I left her and drove home sobbing. This wasn't the process. We knew the risks and took them so she wouldn't be moved around. We rang our social worker and pleaded that she didn't need to go to any other home, we would foster her while grandad got his house ready. We wanted her to have the photographs we had taken, her clothes and toys we had bought. They were hers.

This was the most extraordinary feeling of grief I have ever experienced.

Then came another U-turn, by the evening her paternal grandad had said that he couldn't care for her. He wanted our beautiful baby to have a happy, young home away from his son and to be able to have the start to life she deserves. I will be forever grateful for the enormous decision he made for her. I am heartbroken that he refused all Letterbox contact as I would love to be able to let him know how she is doing; she's having the best life she could have had and we will always love her.

(Hannah and Claire, Foster to Adopt/Fostering for Adoption, girl, one week old)

U-turns are common and adopters are very much bound to the system and the decisions that are being made in the best interests of the child. Sadly, of course, there are those cases where 'the baby/child goes back' (a common phrase that worries most prospective adopters). During our training we heard of one case in our agency, where the decision was made six weeks post-placement. This scared Will and I; being in our agency, it felt closer to home. In responding to the call for case studies, Sarah and Alex were also keen to share their story, their experience of a terminated placement.

We were offered another relinquished baby, he was born prematurely. When we 'got the call' I was in the middle of a meeting at work. I just had to say, *'I have got to go, a baby has been born.'* Within a few hours we were with him in hospital, in intensive care.

For us, the risks associated with a relinquished baby were not as much as a baby who had been exposed to drugs or alcohol. The anxiety with a relinquished baby comes from the wait, where the birth parents can change their mind any time up to the Adoption Order. All through the pregnancy this baby wasn't wanted; birth mother wanted an abortion at 27 weeks, but it was too late. It was at this point she made the decision to place the baby for adoption from birth.

The nurses were amazing. We built such a close relationship with them; they called us mummy and daddy from the moment we met her. It was our tenth wedding anniversary that week; we were there

24 hours a day, doing shifts. The nurses made us a little card which said *'To Mummy and Daddy, Happy 10th Wedding Anniversary'* – they also made a little book for him and put a photograph of us in it. At the time I was worried about this, just in case birth mother changed her mind. She wanted to meet us but the social worker said no for the first two days; they thought she needed time at home to settle.

On the following Tuesday we got a missed call. I had been in the shower, it was a phone number from the area the hospital was in. Then the social worker called me. The phone call that we will never, ever, forget – *'I am really sorry she has changed her mind'* – I just didn't have any words, I put the phone down.

You hear about it, you are asked about it at your panel *'what would you do if the baby went back'* – they are going back to their birth parents so you have to take that as a comfort because that, hopefully, is best for the baby. It was still very hard. It probably will be hard for a long time.

I was just so angry with how we were treated. The allocated social worker, the one who we had spent a lot of time with, dropped off the face of the earth. We had bought the baby so much, we wanted him to have it. There were also items we had left with him in hospital – knitted items from our parents for the baby. There was also a blanket that was very special to us. We had it when we started trying to conceive over ten years ago – we wanted it back. I messaged the social worker the day after, but we didn't hear from her. The nurse rang me to see how we were, I broke down. She kindly sent us back the blankets with a lovely little note. There was another blanket that had been in Alex's family for 20 years, we haven't had that one back. You hear about it happening, but actually going through it is terrible.

I am a great believer in, if it is not meant to be, then it is not meant to be. You have to think like that with Fostering for Adoption. The thing that hurt me the most was my nephew. He was so excited; we had been allowed to video call him with the baby from the hospital. After it happened, he was so sad. I said to him *'we just have to be happy because he is with his mummy'* – that is all I could say, we were broken.

(Sarah and Alex, Foster to Adopt, matching phase)

There is another story I feel is important to share with you. The case study provided by Paul and John shows that in their situation, it was the Local Authority that decided more evidence was needed as to why the baby couldn't stay with their birth family – there needed to be a re-assessment. Sadly for Paul and John, they cared for the baby for three months while the assessments and court proceedings were underway and ultimately they had to say goodbye to the little boy that they had fallen in love with. This is their story.

When we were called about a baby with an EPP, we were reassured that his birth parents were not contesting the plan of adoption and a negative viability assessment had been completed with a birth family member. On this basis we agreed to accept the baby. We met him two days later and fell in love. Our natural instincts kicked in; we were responsible for this child. We looked after him for a week in hospital while he was at the end of drug withdrawal and then took him home. A week later we had another call from our social worker telling us that a manager in the Local Authority didn't think that the viability assessment had been robust enough and they felt that the birth family weren't being given a fair chance to keep the baby.

Our hearts sank, we knew that was the beginning of the end and that ultimately this baby was going to be removed from us. We then had the worst two and a half months of our lives. Contact with the birth family member began as part of a Special Guardianship assessment; we had to hand him over to people we had never met. We wanted to protect him.

We had weeks where formally the decision hadn't been made but everyone knew what the outcome was going to be. Three days after the ADM decision he left us. At the same time John's mother had just passed away and he was out of the country; as a family we were grieving. The day our little one left us was the most horrific day of my life – I remember every detail of the morning he was collected. The social worker arrived and while she gathered up his belongings, I carried him around the house. When she was ready to go, she took him from me at the doorstep. I shut the door and broke down.

(Paul and John, Early Permanence Placement, boy aged two weeks)

For Paul and John, this was devastating. For us, hearing about these cases made it difficult to trust that everything was going to be okay. Right up to the Adoption Order, we found it hard to relax, not knowing if it would work out in the end. For Nick and Louise, they felt that accepting a relinquished baby would be more straightforward, but in the case study below they document the rollercoaster of a ride they had; it was far from a given that this little baby would remain with them:

> Bringing our baby girl home from the hospital was amazing. After ten weeks of near silence from the agency after approval, we had a phone call about a two-day-old baby left in a nearby hospital. Twenty-four hours later we were on our way to pick her up. She was beautiful.
>
> We expected adoption with a relinquished child to be relatively straight forward, but in our case there were bumps in road that brought us perilously close to losing her months into the placement.
>
> Babies can only be relinquished after a minimum of six weeks when a guardian must witness the forms before it becomes legal. This is an anxious period because birth mother can change her mind at any point. We had to wait eight weeks and we were holding our breath the whole time. Caring for a newborn and dealing with the stress of these circumstances was emotionally draining.
>
> In the early days a strong bond formed between us and this gorgeous girl and our boys loved her too. The social workers weren't able to register her birth initially because the registrar wanted to give birth mother more time, in case she wanted to name her. After much uncertainty we were able to go along with the social worker to register her and we were thankful to have this opportunity. Our baby girl was named by a senior social worker.
>
> Our first LAC Review was after one month. The independent reviewing officer (IRO) needed clarification that the embassy of birth mother's nationality had been informed of the situation. They responded that they wanted details of birth mother and wider family to conduct their own investigation. This caused a great deal of stress for all involved. The baby's social worker was very much against their involvement

and birth mother was similarly insistent that her details were not passed on. We were in no way prepared for having to deal with this level of uncertainty.

There were also concerns about her birth father. Birth mother was against the birth father being informed of the birth; he was unaware he had a child. The IRO wanted birth father to be informed, regardless of these wishes, and for him to be given the option of caring for the child. This was yet another period of anxiety as we waited for news.

As Fostering for Adoption carers we were not invited to any meetings about these concerns. After four months of uncertainty the decision was reached to apply for a hearing that would enable the court to decide. This hearing was eventually convened three months later. This was so stressful, there was real threat that we could lose this little girl. Our social workers were all adamant that the decision would almost certainly be in our favour, but as we know going through the process, the unexpected can always happen.

Then the tables turned again. The judge criticised the agency for taking so long to get to this stage and wanted statements from all involved, including from birth mother to explain why birth father shouldn't be contacted. The social worker at this stage voiced that she was concerned that her reasons wouldn't be strong enough. A second hearing was booked for two months later. We were mentally preparing ourselves for losing our little girl and were thinking of how we would approach this with the boys.

Before the second hearing, the guardian managed to convince birth mother to contact birth father herself. He was in a bad place and wasn't interested in caring for a baby or being involved. While this is a sad part of her story, it was a huge relief for us.

On hearing this, the IRO felt that birth father should be given more time to process this news. An ultimatum letter was sent to him, but no reply was received. Finally, three weeks later the IRO signed off the plan for adoption. Our little girl was 11 months old and finally we could breathe.

Our Relinquishment Panel and the Matching Panel followed smoothly and now, at 13 months, we have just submitted our application to adopt.

(Louise and Nick, Foster to Adopt, girl, two days old)

These cases show the everyday realities of Fostering for Adoption – from the last-minute decisions to changed plans, to being on the cusp of losing the little one that has come into your life, and of course for some, having to say goodbye. In accepting an EPP this is what families are agreeing to – being there for the child, no matter what the outcome.

11 October

Every day this week we have been on standby. We have had multiple texts and phone calls from the social workers telling us that various processes need to happen before getting an emergency court hearing. It has really begun to feel like that paperwork has been sitting on someone's desk for all of these weeks. We understand that the process is complex and there are lots of stages to go through but we really feel that we have borne the brunt of poor communication. It just doesn't make sense, there must be commonalities in the process. When we are told that they are *'waiting for an emergency court hearing'* well what does that mean, what is involved, is it an email, are letters sent by post? Does it take a day, a week, a month? We have no idea. When you don't know the system this is a really hard process to navigate. Essentially we are now three weeks on from being told that the placement would be imminent.

Late this afternoon the manager of our agency emailed. She told us that there is a court date booked for 17 October. We had hoped that this would be sooner, but now we are at least grateful that we have a date to work towards. Of course, this is only if the judge agrees with the Fostering for Adoption placement.

This weekend we will have to return the baby clothes we bought a few weeks ago. We were optimistic and had bought 3–6 months outfits; it is much more likely now that we are going to be needing 6–9 months. At least having a date for court gives us a bit of clarity with work.

13 October

I am sitting in a tent with the rain pouring down. We decided that we needed an impromptu few nights away walking in Wales. Despite the weather, the forecast for tomorrow is set to be glorious. We have spent this evening being entertained in a local pub by a Welsh voice choir. I have said it before, but this really better be our last mini trip away without a baby.

14 October

Another sting in the tail. We found out today that our case in court has been double-booked – fortunately, the new date is only a few more days to wait; they have moved it to 23 October. We also had more clarity on the emergency court hearing process – as there is no emergency as such, the court won't grant a sooner hearing – he is safe where he is. We really wish we had been told this weeks ago and not raised our expectations.

With the latest news and the new court date, my boss has asked me to travel abroad to assist my colleagues. I have said I will go but I need to fly home on 22 October. There is no way I can be in another country waiting for news of the court decision to come through. If it all goes to plan I need to be at home to put final preparations in place for introductions to start the next day and if it is disappointing news, equally, I don't want to be away from home.

18 October

I am now away on business. I have again brought Bunny with me for comfort. This is a big week and I need all the comfort I can get. Perhaps by the end of the week he will be sleeping in the arms of our little one, who knows.

22 October

I was able to do a bit of shopping today in between my meetings. I have bought him some gorgeous wooden toys and a few clothes. When I got back to the hotel I showed my colleagues; they are so excited for us. Now that my meetings are over, the nerves are really setting in. While chatting to my colleagues I had missed three calls from the social worker. I really panicked; I was sure that something must have gone wrong. I found a quiet spot in the Reception and rang her back. Thank goodness, she was just checking that we were both okay, no dramas to report this time. Our social worker is amazing. The team have decided that if all goes well tomorrow she will support us with the transition and then once the child has been placed she will hand over to her colleague. I think this is a good decision; we really feel like we need her to get us through the next few days. She told us to sit tight and she would speak to us tomorrow after the court hearing.

My colleagues were waiting for an update and with a beaming smile I told them that there was no panic and all was still on for tomorrow. I had a few hours to pack my bags, say goodbye to my colleagues and head to the airport. It was very strange to say goodbye, thinking that this may be the last time I see them for over a year – if all goes to plan my Adoption Leave will start at the end of this week.

I am now sitting on the plane waiting for take-off and thinking through the three potential scenarios that could happen tomorrow. The first is that the judge will agree with the plan for Fostering for Adoption and transition will begin the day after. Second, the judge turns down the plan for Fostering for Adoption and instead decides on a plan for regular adoption, in which case we would have to wait a few months for the Matching Panel and placement. The third scenario is that something else entirely happens and the plan for this little baby changes. Of course, scenario one is the one we are all hoping for. I am signing out now, making the flight home to hopefully become a mummy.

23 October

Written in the morning

You wouldn't believe what happened last night. Who would have thought I would have ended up in the middle of a security drama at the airport. The flight had been delayed and we were sitting on the plane ready to taxi, every ten minutes or so came more news about further delays. Soon there were rumours about a major security breach and increasingly anxious passengers. Fortunately the whole thing was a false alarm and after an hour and a half our flight took off. I certainly didn't need that last night. Will collected me from the airport and we were home by 11pm.

I didn't have much sleep, tossing and turning, going over the three potential scenarios that could play out. Once I did get to sleep I had a terrible dream, actually a nightmare. I was trying to comfort a baby and just didn't know what to do, he wouldn't go to sleep. I woke up feeling sick – how are we going to know how to get him to sleep? How does he like to be held? What comforts him? My rational, awake self, now thinks – let's get through today first and then worry about how he likes to sleep.

It is six weeks since we heard about this baby boy. This has not only been the hardest phase of the process to date but I would probably say the emotional toil and uncertainty has meant that this is certainly one of the most challenging times of my life. We have talked about this baby, dreamt about him; we have prepared for him, bought him things, taken things back, bought bigger things – we just can't wait any longer. I am so scared that we are going to be let down again and I don't think I can cope with it. I just really want him in our lives. We have been told that cases in court normally begin at 10am and if we haven't heard by 5pm *'not to worry too much'* (I will be climbing the walls if this is the case). They have said that we absolutely will hear the outcome because if introductions are happening tomorrow a plan needs to be put in place.

Written in the evening

Just after 1pm we had 'the call' – the one which confirmed that it was a unanimous decision. This little baby boy is to be adopted and we can start the Fostering for Adoption process tomorrow. It is the best outcome we could have hoped for and we are very fortunate. The judge has granted the Care Order and the Placement Order, meaning that this will be a 'less risky' Fostering for Adoption placement. We can't believe it; this is beyond our expectation and just brilliant. The judge agreed that introductions should begin tomorrow and then over the period of a week he will transition into our home. Three final contact sessions have been ordered between little one and his birth mother. Halfway through the week, there will be a review meeting and if all parties agree, the placement will continue and he will move into our home.

We have been told to bring the soft toy that we have been sleeping with – our Bunny. At 12 noon tomorrow, in less than 24 hours, we will meet our little one. Typing this is overwhelming; this is it, we can finally be excited.

In the run-up to the court hearing there was no mention of potentially a Placement Order being granted, so we were delighted when we heard this news. However, given that it was a Fostering for Adoption placement we were still cautious about the potential outcome. Our social workers explained that for various reasons Fostering for Adoption placements can be granted post-Placement Order (indeed, as in our case). The extract below is useful in explaining the legalities of this:

> [T]here are occasionally situations in which local authorities find that they need to place a child with their prospective adopters after the Placement Order has been made but before the Matching Panel. In these cases, approved adopters can be given temporary approval under Reg 25A. Possible situations could include where a child has to make an immediate move from their short-term foster placement before the adoption match can be made and there is an identified need to avoid further placement moves for the child, or where the Foster for Adoption placement is being made because there has been a challenge from a birth family member to the Placement Order but there is a desire to prevent future delay in the child's move. In the latter situation, the prospective carers would need to be made very aware of the potential of the court to return the child to the birth parent.
>
> (Dibben and Howorth, 2017, p 18)

CHAPTER 6

OUR STORY FEELS REAL: TRANSITION AND PLACEMENT

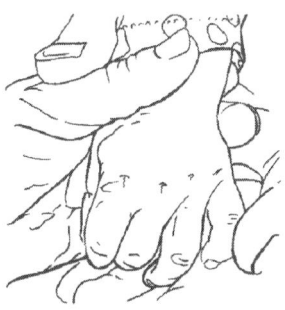

In this chapter we meet our little one for the first time. We have an amazing, emotional transition week, where we take our first steps in caring for him, and we sign paperwork to say we will take responsibility of him on a Fostering for Adoption placement. We are nervous, happy, scared and excited.

Here we begin the day after the court decision, the day we meet our little one.

24 October

It is 8am and I can't believe that today is the day. I have now officially finished work. I got up at 4am to send final emails and put on my out of office – that is it, I am now on Adoption Leave. As I type, Will is finishing off his work and then we have a few hours to prepare for a very special journey, to see our baby for the first time. We have wanted this for so long but now the time has arrived I am not really sure what I am meant to be doing. I am feeling a mixture of fear and excitement. I can't wait to meet him, touch him, hold him, but I am also so anxious about it.

We have been instructed to meet the social workers at the foster carers' house at 12 noon. The plan is to have an initial meeting and then to stay at their house until bedtime. Over the next seven days he will transition into our home. We start off with spending a few hours at a time with him, building up over the week to him moving into his new home. This is finally happening.

From this point on I am writing about our transition week retrospectively. At the time I only jotted down a few notes, but this week is firmly etched in memory. As we drove to the foster carers' house (the journey took us just over an hour) we speculated about what kind of house they lived in. We had been told that the family had two children of their own, four others who had recently moved in on a foster placement, our little one and seven dogs. We pulled into their street and nervously counted the numbers on the houses until our eyes locked on the home of our little one. The front door was open and we squinted to see if we could see anyone inside. A lady came to the door, she was mopping the hallway and several children were running between her legs, then the door closed. We were a little early so they were clearly getting ready for our arrival. After a few minutes our social worker arrived and we got out of the car and had a nervous exchange. At the allocated time we rang the doorbell. The door opened, out came the cleaner, a few children and a couple of adults. We stood in the hallway and there were three babies looking up at us. *'Which one was ours?'* I thought.

I looked down to my right, standing with his back to the wall was a little boy, I guessed that he was probably aged one. I then glanced at the foster carer, she was holding a small baby – *'no that can't be him, this baby is too small'* (we later found out that he was three months). My third glance down was to a baby in a bouncer. He looked up at us – *'this must be him, our little boy'.* Sure enough, a few seconds later, he was whipped out of the bouncer and handed to Will, *'Jake, this is your mummy and daddy'.* I couldn't believe it, she actually called us mummy and daddy. My immediate thought was *'that is a bit premature'* – it made me nervous and anxious. I wasn't sure if she should be saying this, given the Fostering for Adoption arrangement.

After a few minutes of standing in the hallway we were ushered into the living room. We sat down on the sofa, Will holding Little Jake – he looked a natural. We spent some time going through the paperwork (although if I am honest it was hard to focus on anything other than the beautiful baby lying in my husband's arms) and we all agreed the timetable for the next few days – as Jake transitions from Jane and David's care to ours. The parting words from the social worker as she left the house were '*you shadow the foster carer for a few days and then gradually take over his care.*' She then said goodbyes and dashed off to another meeting. Jane said, '*Well I haven't got time for that, I've got five other kids to look after – Jake needs his nappy changing.*' Straight in at the deep end.

She laid him down on the mat in the living room and showed us where the nappies, cream and bags were. Fortunately Jake was very compliant; he lay on his back bemused by the flurry of activity in front of him. Jane left us to it and started washing bottles in the kitchen. This one nappy seemed like a herculean effort – which way round? How much cream? How tight? After a few pops back into the kitchen to ask Jane, we were done – we had put on our first nappy, BINGO! Jake then started to cry and Jane appeared in the living room with a syringe of pink fluid, announcing that he had been a bit unwell and should have some medicine.

'*Oh no, our little baby is poorly*' I thought, followed shortly by, '*a syringe, what are we meant to do with that?*'

Will was holding Jake and Jane handed me the syringe. I was so stressed. Out of pure panic I shot the contents of the syringe onto Will's jumper, entirely missing Jake's mouth. What a moment. This learning curve was a little too steep. Little did I know that giving medicine was a common occurrence with teething infants; it really wasn't anything to worry about.

The next few hours passed in a blur. Jake had his afternoon nap, wrapped in a blanket in my arms. We sat on the sofa for 90 minutes while he slept. I couldn't help but shed a tear. Here I was with a baby in my arms – the first time I had properly held him – he was content and asleep, his skin touching mine. We studied his sleeping face, his little nose, long eyelashes and smooth skin, he was beautiful. As we sat familiarising ourselves with his sleeping face, it hit us; this was the baby, our number 8 that needed our care.

Our visit ended at 3:30pm. The plan had originally been to stay until bedtime but Jane didn't want us to meet her girls on Day 1. She thought it would be better for them to meet us tomorrow morning. They were going to tell them tonight that Jake's transition to his new family had started. Due to the unpredictability surrounding placements, they had wanted to wait until they knew for sure that he would be starting transition this week; they are going to be devastated. Before we left, we handed over Bunny; tonight he would be placed in Jake's cot and hopefully he would come to recognise our smell.

We said goodbye to everyone and made the journey to my parents' house to stay the night. On the car journey we beamed from ear to ear, everything could not be more perfect. We had met the most beautiful baby boy, the baby boy we were to care for. We drove away from their house knowing that we had done the right thing; we have made the most amazing decision and this was the start of the next chapter. Whatever happens, we knew from this moment that we would do our very best for him, whatever the outcome. I knew both of our parents would be anxious having not yet heard from us, so I sent them a message: *'Going to stop at the shop to buy nappies ... head over heels in love with him, he is perfect.'*

Staying at my parents' house tonight was a good plan, we have to be back tomorrow morning reasonably early. It was also lovely to be able to share our excitement. When we arrived my parents were so excited but also nervous to hear how it had gone. We decided not to tell them anything and arrange a video call with Will's parents, so we could go through everything together. We both had a quick shower to freshen up and then sat around the kitchen table to share our news. They had lots of questions and over the next hour we retold the ins and outs of the day. One of the first questions they asked was to see a photograph. We hadn't taken any, in the first few hours of meeting him we were so engrossed in taking over his care that we hadn't really thought about it. We were also not sure about the protocol for taking his photograph – were we allowed to? Who can we show it to? Are we allowed to show our parents and friends? Tomorrow we would make sure we ask and hopefully we can show our parents a photograph.

We were told today that we should be wearing the same clothes each day, so he gets used to the sight of us. As we had already packed for the next few days we didn't account for this as it wasn't mentioned in our training session – so my mum put on a load of washing, to make sure we were ready for tomorrow. We had an early night, the exhaustion had kicked in, the adrenaline worn off. We were ready for bed.

Throughout the process you try to imagine this day, the day you meet your baby, your little one. You play it over in your head, over and over, but nothing can prepare you. Standing in the hallway this morning, looking down at those three babies is a moment that will stay with me forever.

I am going to bed with a weight lifted off my shoulders. I now know that we are going to be okay; we can do this. We hugged each other and blew a kiss to our little one in another home, with another loving family. Tonight he will snuggle with Bunny and tomorrow we are one day closer to bringing him home.

25 October

I hardly slept last night, I was far too excited. We had an early start; by 7am we were ringing their doorbell, eager to see him again. The door opened and there he was, in the arms of the foster carer, looking gorgeous in his green sleepsuit. The house was buzzing, there were children everywhere. We were directed into the living room to meet the foster carer's birth children (aged seven and nine); they were apprehensive to meet us. Jake had lived with them since birth; he was very much loved. As soon as the girls saw us they cried. They cried because with us standing in their living room, it was suddenly real, we were going to be taking him away – they were so attached to him. We found out later on that they were also crying out of relief. They liked us, they were relieved that they liked the family that had been chosen for Little J. There were more tears all round as we did introductions. There and then I realised how delicate this situation was for these children. We really needed to manage this transition well, not only for Jake and us, but for these children; this was important.

Similar to Day 1, we started immediately. It was time for his breakfast, followed by his morning nap. David kindly asked if we would like a sausage sandwich. This was very much appreciated. We had been told in the training not to expect food and take your own drinks; some foster carers are happy for you to use their kitchen, others less so. Eating our sausage sandwich with the rest of the family was another icebreaker, making us feel comfortable in their home.

The whole situation is so surreal. You are in a stranger's home and all eyes are on you. They are watching how you pick him up, how you stroke his hand, how you change his nappy, how you make his bottle – there are eyes everywhere. However, despite the eyes, we felt so welcome, they were accommodating and lovely towards us; the crash course in parenting had begun. As the morning progressed, I involved the girls. I asked them questions about him, asked them to help choose his clothes for the day, made sure that they had opportunities to hold and cuddle him. They really love him.

Jane asked if we would like to go out for a coffee. She had arranged for her mum to look after the other children, so she, David, Will and I could go out with the three babies. It took us a while to get Jake ready and leave the house; we wrapped him up warm and put him in his buggy. It felt amazing; we were actually outside, in the real world, with a real baby. We were navigating pavements and ramps and suddenly aware of our environment from the perspective of a parent.

We had a lovely coffee and used the time to ask Jane and David more questions about Jake's routine and his early days. Looking back this is something we hadn't really anticipated, how much they knew about his life. Just as the social workers had given us a detailed account of the decisions which led up to the Fostering for Adoption placement, so too did his foster carers. His story suddenly became alive and real.

When we got back to the house we decided to ask about photographs. Our parents couldn't wait another day; they couldn't wait to see this little baby that one day might be their grandson. We couldn't wait to show them how incredibly beautiful he was. Jane wasn't sure of the official protocol but thought it would be fine for us to take some photographs to show our parents, as long as we don't share them on social media. We would then ask the social workers about the plan for photographs going forward. He lay on the floor with a big beaming smile and we took the first few photographs of our little boy; we will treasure these forever.

It was time to say goodbye. We discussed the plan for tomorrow. Jane suggested that we might like to bring our own baby bag and pram. She said that we needed to start using our own nappies and food. Again, this was something that we hadn't been made aware of on the training, but makes sense in terms of him transitioning into our care. On our way home we sent a few photographs to our parents, their first glimpse of this little baby.

When we got home our first job was to dismantle the cot. As he is now six months old we had set up the cot in his own room. However, he is used to sleeping in the foster carers' room, so we decided that he should be with us for a few months. We have positioned the cot at the end of our bed. I am so excited that he will soon be sleeping in our room.

26 October

It is now the end of Day 3 and we are exhausted. We were grateful for the slightly later start this morning which meant we could get a few jobs done before we left. The foster carers had planned to take us out for lunch. We arrived at 12 noon and soon left the house to walk to their local pub. The family are well known in the community; most people we walked past gave a friendly nod, said hello or stopped to chat. Today the older foster children were being looked after by their friends; the social workers had given permission for this to happen. In Jane's words, *'this week is all about Jake and what is best for him and his new family'* – it is so lovely that they want this week to go as smoothly as possible for us all. We had a lovely lunch together and this now counts as our first meal out with Little J; it went well. A nappy change was needed in the pub and Will offered – both returned unscathed.

We spent the afternoon back at their house, chatting and looking after Jake. The plan was to stay until bedtime. With so many children, understandably bedtime was a bit fluid, so we stayed later than we had initially expected. Tonight was bath and shower night for all the children, so the routine took longer than it would otherwise. It was lovely to see the family in full swing; it was a well-oiled machine. We sat on the sofa, cuddling Jake while hair was plaited, stories read and milk drunk. It is so wonderful to see how much Jane and David love all the children in their care – while plaiting one of the foster children's hair, Jane took the opportunity to speak to her about any worries she was having about her contact session with her birth parent the following day. It was incredible to watch – the sensitivity and love that Jane gave to each of the children was beautiful.

After his bath, Jake fell asleep and we carried him up to bed. It was a little shock to find out that all three babies were sleeping in the same room as Jane and David, there was a cot on each side of the bed and one at the end. Jake's cot was on the other side of the room and it was a little tricky to climb across their bed to put him down; at the same time as not making any noise as the other babies were asleep. As this was our first time, Jane came up with us to show us what to do. She showed us that he loves his teddy touching his face and told us that once his arms are in a relaxed position above his head he is in a deep sleep. He looked so peaceful and calm, just beautiful. By this time it was 9pm so we made a quick exit once he was asleep to give Jane and David some time alone – we are also aware of how exhausting this process must be for them, both physically and emotionally.

We are staying with my parents again. Just as we were dropping off to sleep a message came through on my phone. It was a photograph of Little J asleep in his cot – *'Night, night Mummy and Daddy.'* So kind of Jane to do this, just magical.

27 October

The plan for today was for us to take Jake back to our house for the afternoon. When we arrived at the foster carers' house this morning there was a bit of confusion about logistics. Two of the other foster children now had a contact session arranged with their birth parents which meant that Jane would have to be in multiple places at the same time. Then there was also the issue of the two other babies. Kindly her mum offered to step in and look after the babies. Jane didn't want them coming to our house as well, *'this was Jake's day and special for him and his family.'*

We left at 12 noon to make the journey to our house. I travelled with Jane and Jake, while Will drove ahead in our car. The closer we got the more nervous I became. I really wanted Jane to like our home and feel comfortable. I wanted her to know that Jake is coming to a lovely, happy home. I need not have worried, she was so kind about our house. She said it was *'like being in a spa ... so quiet and calm ... and Jake would love it.'* She acknowledged that it was a world apart from the noise, hustle and bustle of their home. She didn't stay long, just long enough for us to be able to take a few photographs. Before she left she took one of the three of us standing on the doorstep – such a special memory to have. We waved goodbye and closed the door. We couldn't believe it, we had an actual baby in our house. We took him upstairs to show him his room, his little eyes scanned the room and took it all in. It was soon time for his afternoon nap. We rocked him to sleep as Jane had taught us. It is a relatively strong rocking motion, with Bunny touching his face. He soon went to sleep and we put him down in his new cot, at the base of our bed. I can't quite remember how many times I checked him but it was a lot. We pretty much just watched him sleep, in awe of the sleeping baby in our room.

He woke after an hour and a half. After a feed and a nappy change, we decided to take him out for a walk in the pram. We wrapped him up warm and headed off on one of our usual routes. It was a beautiful, crisp, winter afternoon, the sun was shining, life was perfect. While we were out we bumped into our young neighbour; he was out for a walk with his grandparents. These were the first people in the village to officially meet our baby. There were tears in their eyes; they were so pleased for us which was so touching. Soon after we bumped into another lady, someone we don't really know. After meeting him she said, *'Oh you need to get inside, the fog is bad for babies.'* Our first experience of parental advice from the sidelines – we had no idea fog was bad for babies. We headed back home walking slightly faster, just in case.

Before we knew it, it was bath time. We had done this once at Jane's house so knew his routine. He loved splashing in the water and his post-bath snuggles. Once we had wrapped him up in his pyjamas we put him in the car seat and made the return journey back to the foster carers' house. At the other end we gave him his bottle before putting him to bed. We had a quick chat with Jane and David before heading home again. It has been a brilliant day. We really feel like we are taking over his care, making decisions for him and getting to know his routines and quirks.

28 October

Before leaving last night we were told that Jake would be going to a contact session with his birth mother in the morning. The new plan was for us to arrive at the foster carers' house by 1:30pm in time for our mid-way review meeting. This was to check that everyone was happy with how the transition was going and to confirm the plan going forward.

Mid-morning we had a text from Jane to say that the contact session had not taken place, birth mother had not turned up, so when we were ready we could head over. My reaction to this news surprised me. I was sad. I was upset that she hadn't turned up; this was the penultimate session with her baby. Perhaps it was just too much for her to cope with.

The wider team were at the foster carers' house for the transition meeting. There were a few other adults in the house (family and friends of the foster carers), so they were ushered into the kitchen so that our meeting could take place in the living room, away from the other foster children and prying ears. It was relatively quick and a massive relief to hear that everyone was happy and that the transition for Little J was going well. Once again there were a few tears from Jane and myself – it is all just so overwhelming. I am beginning to feel the loss that Jane and her family are experiencing.

After the meeting, Jane suggested that Will and I take Jake into town for a coffee, our first mini trip out with him on our own. We had brought our own buggy and his new winter snowsuit – it is navy and white striped – he looks beautiful in it. We strapped him into the pram and off we went, on our own, an adventure into town. After a few photographs en route and both of us 'having a go' at pushing the pram, we decided that a celebratory coffee and cake was in order. It felt good but I did feel like all eyes were on us. I felt like everyone else knew that we were new to this game, it made me anxious. This time it was my turn for the nappy change, and I did it, all on my own; proud is an understatement. After our coffee and a quick browse around a few shops we decided to head back. We hadn't agreed with Jane how long we were allowed to be out for, so thought we best return. Technically the responsibility for Jake was still with Jane, so we didn't want her to be worrying about where we were.

This afternoon we had more texts from friends and family asking for his name and photographs of him. We discussed this with the social workers during our meeting. Until the responsibility for Jake has been transferred from the foster carer to us we can't share any details. Once we have responsibility for him we can share his name and a photograph with close friends and family. However, we have to be clear that they can't forward the message on to others and most certainly no images on social media. We are happy that we now know the protocol for this and look forward to sending a message to our nearest and dearest in a few days.

We gave him a bath and his bottle and stayed until he went to sleep. He is being so patient with us which is just amazing.

29 October

Today has been our longest day taking care of Jake. We arrived at the foster carers' house by 6:30am in time to give him his morning bottle. I still haven't got the hang of making bottles – there is so much to think about, from using their oven to boil the water, measuring out the formula, what we can touch and not touch (due to the sterilising) and then working out if the milk is too hot or not warm enough. Our little one is very particular about the temperature of his milk. A few months ago the foster carers went on holiday for two weeks, so Jake went into respite care with another foster family. He came back with a few new habits – one that he needed a dummy to settle, having never had one before, and second that he now liked his milk a little warmer than usual. First thing this morning we experienced this first-hand. I had made the bottle and he flatly refused it. He was letting us know that he was hungry but wouldn't take the milk. Jane popped her head round the door to see what was going on. She simply said, *'It isn't hot enough ... it needs to be warmer than that.'* Sure enough, after a few more minutes of the milk standing in the boiling water, he was happy with the temperature. Spot on for Little J; he finished the whole bottle.

After his bottle and with Jake still in his pyjamas we got in the car and headed back to our house for the day. Once home we spent the day working through his routine, ticking off the sleep, eat, tummy time, repeat – it was important to do this to make him feel safe and secure. The only thing we decided to change was to put him to sleep in his cot, rather than on us. We put him in a sleeping bag, closed the blind and let him have a proper sleep in our room. After two hours, he was still asleep. From what Jane had told us, he never sleeps for that long. We started to worry. I decided to text her and ask her what to do, leave him or wake him? Her response sent us into a mild panic. She asked us to check his temperature to see if he was unwell. Our instinct told us that he wasn't unwell, but now she has said it, why was he still asleep? The next drama was that our new thermometer didn't have any batteries. We texted a neighbour who came straight over with one to borrow. We woke him, checked his temperature and he was fine. Panic over. He probably slept for longer because he was exhausted with all of the change and he was enjoying some peace and quiet.

Today has been quite stressful. I have felt panicked about looking after Jake correctly. After checking his temperature we also thought he sounded a bit chesty. While he was asleep he also scratched himself with his fingernail.

When we spotted it I was upset. I am paranoid about any marks or scratches on him in fear of what the social workers will think. Will is much more rational about this, but I am very anxious.

Tonight we gave him a bath and headed back to the foster carers house to put him to bed. After settling him for the night we drove back home. We need a few hours tomorrow morning to get the house ready for his arrival the following day. Thank goodness we had prepared some meals; we are too exhausted to think about cooking. We are exhausted with learning how to be parents, exhausted with the travelling, exhausted with being in an intense situation with the foster carers and emotionally exhausted with the enormity of what we were doing.

30 October

Before we left yesterday evening Jane suggested that we should take Jake to the doctor to get his chest checked; she was keen that we get the reassurance that he is okay before he moves in with us tomorrow. We agreed this was a good idea.

We woke up this morning to another issue; it had rained heavily overnight and our village had flooded. We were busy getting the house ready and Jane texted me at 9:30am to say she had managed to get an appointment with the doctor at 11am. As it takes just over an hour to get there, we quickly had to pack our overnight bags, sort out Jake's clothes, bottles and bags and bundle everything into the car as fast as we could. The flooding and road closures made for a stressful journey.

We arrived and headed straight to the doctors; it was a ten-minute drive. The appointment went really well, and the doctor was lovely. She gave him a thorough check and reassured us that he would be fine. We explained that we are taking over his care and she gave us a crash course in what to look out for: rashes, temperature and breathing. Despite doing an infant first aid course, having a baby in front of us was a different matter. It was lovely of the doctor to be so empathetic to our situation. She wished us well and we left feeling confident that he was going to be alright.

The rest of today was busy. While Jake was sleeping, Jane and I went through all of his clothes. She said that we could take any of them home with us. She was keen to tell us that Jake has his own special clothes. The more she talked about him, I knew she was in love. Jake was their first foster baby and their bond was strong; he was very special to all of them. There were some clothes she wanted to give me for his memory box, including the outfit that he came to her from hospital in and the babygrow she had bought for him when they went on their family holiday. Will and I went through the piles and piles of clothes and chose the ones to take home. We were aware of not taking too many, as there were other foster babies living with them. Jane also told us that she would be sending him with his baby monitor, his bath toys and of course his dummy. The social workers were keen for us to take as many of his belongings today, to avoid us doing this tomorrow, the final day – there is to be no lingering as departure needs to be as swift as possible.

As the afternoon progressed we began to feel the tiredness and exhaustion kick in. It has been a long week and we really wanted to be back in our home with Jake. Mid-afternoon I started to feel sick and had an unsettled stomach. I wasn't sure if it was caused by something I had eaten or if the anxiety about tomorrow was building.

The plan was for us all to have dinner together. We asked the children what they would like to eat and they chose fish and chips. Will and I treated everyone to say thank you to the family. It was lovely to be all able to eat together but the tension was building. As it drew closer to bedtime the girls were getting visibly upset. This was their last night with Jake; they gave him drawings for his memory box and lots of cuddles.

This was hard for Jane to see. These were her children getting upset about Jake leaving; it was tough for them all, it was emotional. We had hoped that tonight we would get him settled and then have an early night ahead of our big day tomorrow but it didn't quite go to plan. We didn't leave until 10pm. By 8:30pm he was asleep but unfortunately one of the other babies in the room was unsettled so woke him up; at 9:30pm we were rocking him back to sleep. It was a long and emotional day.

As we left the house and drove to my parents' house we couldn't help but be relieved that today was the last transition day; we were ready to bring him home. We had a quick chat over a cup of tea with my parents and then headed to bed. We were utterly exhausted.

Before going to sleep I wrote a card to give to Jane and David tomorrow:

Dear Jane and David,

Thank you so much for giving us the most amazing transition week with Jake.

In one week we have learnt so much about how to care for him, his needs and routines. It has been brilliant and we are confident that we now have the basic blocks to build on.

I am sure you know it already but J is going to be loved so much. We have been on a very long, tough journey to get to this stage and finally we can get excited about taking over his care.

You are both wonderful human beings, the love, generosity and warmth you give to each of the children in your care is second to none.

I am sure that Jake is going to leave a hole in your lives, but let's not be sad that it's over, but be excited about what is to come. Once we are settled into our new life we will arrange to meet.

Thank you so much for giving Jake the best beginning, we hope that this is the start of our life as a family of three.

Alice and Will

31 October

I hardly slept a wink last night. I cried and cried. Writing the card to Jane and David made me terribly sad; my heart ached for the loss they were about to endure. I wasn't nervous, I was 100 per cent sure this little baby was the right match for us; neither of us had any concerns. All my feelings were directed towards someone else's loss. Today they had to say goodbye to a baby they had supported when he was most vulnerable, a baby they had loved from day one.

We were up early, puffy eyes and anxious about the day ahead (I say we here, but really I mean me, Will was his usual calm self). We had breakfast with my parents but I could hardly eat, I felt sick. Before we left, my mum took a photograph of us on their front doorstep, our last photograph as a couple before we became a three. I was teary; not only did I still feel poorly but I was cross and upset that I felt ill. I wanted more than anything for this day to be perfect. Our final meeting was scheduled for 10am, planned to be calm and swift. Jane had arranged for her mum to also be there to give her support once we had left. Jake's social worker was already there when we arrived and Jake was ready to go. He had been dressed in the 'going home' outfit that we had prepared for him yesterday and there was a small bag of belongings including his baby monitor, Bunny and blanket.

Standing in the living room, before our final goodbye I asked if we could have a photograph together to show Little J one day. This was the end of our transition week and the start of the next chapter. Within ten minutes we were strapping Jake into his car seat and waving to Jane and her mum standing on the doorstep. This was it, time to take Jake home.

I sat with him in the back of the car and held his hand. He was soon asleep, soothed by the vibrations of the car. He woke as we entered our village, his village. We unloaded the car and brought him into the house in his car seat. He looked so small, looking up at us on the floor in the living room. More tears flowed as Will and I hugged.

I still felt terrible, so we decided that I should go to bed for a sleep. I was no use to Will or Jake feeling like this. I drew the blind in the bedroom, pulled over the duvet cover and fell fast asleep for two hours. When I woke I felt a bit better. Will was on top of it all; he had made the lunch, the washing was on, Jake was fed and soon due his nap. At 2pm we had the scheduled visit from Jake's social worker. After giving us a few hours to settle she was coming to check that we were okay and to complete the paperwork. This was to transfer responsibility for Jake from the foster carers to us. Now the documents have been signed we have joint responsibility for him, with the Local Authority.

The social worker went through a whole series of rules and processes to follow. During the fostering stage we need to keep a logbook of everything that Jake does, for example, what he has eaten, drunk, any medication, where he has been and how he has slept. A copy of this needs to be sent to our social workers on a weekly basis. If we want to stay overnight somewhere with him we need to email or text our social workers with the name and full address of where we are going. Overnight stays are not usually permitted within the first three months of placement. She also pointed out the obvious restrictions, such as children in your care not being able to have piercings (!) and no adventurous activity. By this she meant climbing mountains – which she felt she needed to emphasise to us given our adventurous streak. We also talked through what we should do in an emergency. If there was a medical emergency, then obviously we would call the appropriate emergency services. Jake has a red flag on his record identifying a Looked After Child, so they would know to call his allocated social worker. They also advised that we contact our social workers and the duty officer. What was said next shocked us, we were told *'if birth parents turn up at your door then ring the police immediately.'* I hadn't even considered that this might be a potential scenario; how would they know where we live?

During our training we were told that we should not have visitors within the first three weeks, not even our parents. We were surprised to hear the social worker ask when our parents were coming to meet Little J – was this a test? We tentatively replied *'tomorrow.'* Her response *'I am glad to hear it, you can tell Jake is happy and content and I am sure you will introduce him to people in the way you feel appropriate for him.'* What a relief.

Once the social worker left we were soon aware that we had not updated any of our friends and family; we hadn't even let our parents know that we were home and all was well. I checked my phone and we had dozens of lovely messages. Late afternoon we decided it was time to make an official announcement. Earlier in the week we had drafted some messages for Facebook and WhatsApp. We spent some time tweaking the messages and deciding which photographs to send to people. The social workers had agreed that we could send a photograph of him to our friends and family via WhatsApp (asking them not to distribute further) and then use an anonymous photograph for Facebook.

What we didn't anticipate were the hundreds of replies which immediately followed our announcement. It was overwhelming and emotional; everyone was so happy for us. This finally felt real, after all these years of waiting, hoping and praying, we were announcing that we had a baby in our family, how amazing. We took in the moment and spent some time cuddling Little J before starting the bedtime routine.

We read him a new book we had been given, it ended:

> Our kisses are colours, and raindrops that flow, and pebbles, and acorns, and comets that glow, and flowers, and snowflakes that fall from above; they're our way, sweet baby to give you our love.
>
> (Lawler, 2011)

As Jake lay in Will's arms and I read the story my voice started to wobble, and a tear rolled down my cheek. This was it, the beginning.

He went to sleep like a dream; like us, he was probably completely exhausted.

CHAPTER 7

DOCUMENTING THE DETAIL OF OUR STORY: THE EARLY DAYS OF FOSTERING FOR ADOPTION

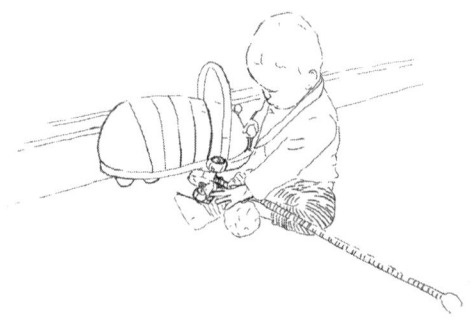

Here I document the early days, the ins and outs of our Fostering for Adoption placement. For us, the first few weeks were purely about survival. Being launched into parenthood and being closely monitored by social services was intense. Learning to look after a baby was the hardest thing we have ever done. The tiredness, emotion, and love were all punctuated with uncertainty.

1 November

We had a good first night, we only had to get up a few times to check him. He is a noisy sleeper; it was nice to be able to hear his heavy breathing as we lay in bed listening. He woke early, 5am, so Will and I took it in turns to have cuddles on the sofa downstairs. I felt so much better; after a good night's sleep I was feeling refreshed. It felt like Christmas morning, with a buzz of excitement and anticipation in the air. We had a lovely relaxing morning, doing a few jobs and getting into his routine of feeding, playing and sleeping.

Will's parents arrived late afternoon for tea; it was so lovely to see them. They had brought flowers, cards and a cake embossed with the letter J, just perfect. He was so calm and took it all totally in his stride. We are so pleased that we made the decision to introduce him to our parents early on; they have been with us on this journey every step of the way and we couldn't imagine them not being able to see him this weekend. I must emphasise though that we only made this decision as our social worker encouraged us to, given how content and happy Jake had been over the course of the transition process. If there had been any sign of him being unsettled then meeting our parents in the early days would have been delayed.

Later on in the afternoon we went for a walk around the block with Jake in the pram. Soon after we had this wonderful message from one of our neighbours:

> So my spies tell me that you've been perambulating the streets today with an actual perambulator with an actual boy inside ... I am so happy for you both ... beamingly so.

It is so lovely to have such wonderful friends, who know how special this time is for us.

2 November

Today was the turn of my parents to visit, such a special day. Jake again was an absolute star. I can tell they love him already – they are besotted with him. I can't wait to see their relationship blossom, as grandparents and grandchild – although thoughts such as this are tainted with the uncertainty of the Fostering for Adoption process; we have all got to hope that this little one will stay with us forever. The weather was lovely this afternoon, a crisp winter's day. We wrapped up and went for a walk, a family walk, all of us together. My parents had come laden with presents from friends and family. We had a cup of tea and sat opening the gifts, from rattles to books, baby clothes, vouchers and more. We can't believe how generous people are being – the thank you list has begun.

During the training, we were told that limited contact with friends and family is needed in the early days of placement, to ensure that the child becomes familiar and feels safe with their new family. The more I speak to adopters and Fostering for Adoption carers, the more I see that this really has to be assessed on a case-by-case basis. For us, Jake was settled and content and with the social worker's permission, our parents were able to meet him for an hour or so in the first few days. One of the ironic aspects of the adoption process is that you spend so long justifying the support you have around you, only to find that you have to limit contact with your support network in the early days. I have spoken to newly placed adopters who are fragile, emotional and desperately need the support of their parents to get through this time. For us, we couldn't imagine not sharing this special moment with them. In the case study below, Rachel describes how she kept her little boy's familiar routines and smells to make sure he felt safe and secure.

> We spent two weeks at home together and only went out for his contact sessions with birth family. We had a small number of visits from immediate family and my best friend during this time, but I made sure that I was providing all of his comfort and personal care, so that he wasn't being held by lots of new people. He arrived with several vests, babygrows and a couple of blankets. I dressed him in each of these outfits over the next few days before dressing him in anything washed with my washing powder, trying to keep some familiarity for him. He used his blanket for several weeks before it desperately needed washing.
> (Rachel, Foster to Adopt, boy, six weeks)

Of course in the early days of placement many families have to not only get used to caring for a new baby but also work the logistics of contact into their routine and life. Louise and Ian share their experience of contact sessions with their three-month-old little girl. They explain that they were their child's advocate during the process:

> Poppy came to us in late 2019 at nine weeks old on a Fostering for Adoption placement via our Local Authority. An Interim Care Order had been sought after birth. At the time of the move, family links had already been ruled out but further detailed assessments of the birth parents were required before the social workers returned to court for a Placement Order. Prior to Poppy being placed we knew that we would be facilitating contact with her birth family, three times a week for two hours a time. Twice a week with the birth mother and once a week with the birth father.

Once Poppy moved in with us contact resumed within a couple of days. Arrangements were made with contact supervisors who determined the place and time. This was a closed Fostering for Adoption placement which meant that we couldn't take Poppy to a contact centre, we had to meet contact workers in various places, such as supermarket car parks.

Initially while we were both on leave, we made sure that we had something to do during the contact session and that we both went to the handover point. When this was no longer feasible, I tended to stay within a 5–10 minute drive of the handover point as we had several instances of birth parents not attending contact or turning up late.

We were quite anxious when Poppy was at contact and it was important that we talked about it with each other and our social worker. We had to live with the fact that we were in limbo and contact was part of this process. We had a few instances of miscommunication, usually about stand-in contact supervisors, and on more than one occasion, we were kept waiting at the handover point. It was up to us to make sure that Poppy was comfortable and happy – we had to be her advocate during this process.

(Louise and Ian, Foster to Adopt, girl, three months)

Elaine and James also share their experience of contact with both of their babies (for context they are in Northern Ireland). They explain how much involvement they had with a diverse range of professionals, the logistics surrounding contact and how for their baby the contact sessions became too distressing and so the team made the decision that Elaine would also attend.

Both our little ones came to us very early (seven weeks old and seven days old) on a Concurrent Care Placement. Both had two or three weekly contact visits, often early mornings with birth parents an hour's drive away from our home. We had to be available for social worker visits once a fortnight, LAC Reviews every six weeks, medical appointments with the Local Authority appointed doctors (ours was a four-hour round trip) and visits from the guardian (an independent person acting solely in the interest of the little ones).

For our first little one, contact was three times a week which very quickly reduced to twice to help birth parents (mostly birth mother) engage. It was sporadic at best, sometimes we turned up and then were told that it was cancelled. After about three months our little one started to get distressed with the contact sessions; the supervising social worker and the social worker team decided it would be best if I was also present. It was a little awkward at first but it was valuable time for both of us and we got to know a little about the birth family (likes and dislikes, family, school, sports) – important information for our little one's life story book.

At times, it felt that all the disruption was not in the best interests of a tiny baby and we were certainly asked to do more than a parent with a 'child of their own' would have to do. That said, our social workers went out of their way to help and support us.

(Elaine and James, Concurrent Placement from birth, a sibling to their three year-old)

Organising the logistics of contact can be particularly hard when there are multiple children involved. For Charlotte and Richard, one child had contact and the other one didn't which meant that one of them had to stay at home and look after 'Big Brother' while the other took 'Little Brother' to contact visits. For them, they also found themselves in a position where they were having face-to-face contact with the birth family. In the extract below they describe how emotional this was for them. This combined with all the daily responsibilities, the permissions and the anxiety around emergency hospital visits was stressful and exhausting.

We had contact with birth family 2–3 times per week. We found this particularly challenging due to the many face-to-face interactions we had. To see firsthand the loss, trauma and grief that they were experiencing was difficult to navigate emotionally. Contact involved three hours of travelling and one of us needed to be at home to look after Big Brother as he had already completed his final contact with birth family. On top of this we had numerous other responsibilities including: daily records, monthly health visitor visits, social worker visits every 5–6 weeks for both children, LAC Reviews and medicals – this was all very time consuming. In the first few months, Little Brother was very ill and he spent time in hospital. This was very worrying and at this time we were giving daily health updates to the social worker.

The rules on leaving the boys in the care of others were very vague. From our understanding it is a grey area and it depends on your Local Authority, the child's social worker and the individual case. For us, the boy's Local Authority was strict, so at all times they remained in our care.

All of this was a lot to deal with, on top of finding our way as new parents and building attachment to Big Brother, who had experienced so much trauma and loss during his first year of life.
(Charlotte and Richard, Foster to Adopt, siblings, weeks apart, one from foster care and a baby from hospital)

Of course the contact sessions may mean that Fostering for Adoption carers meet the birth parents in both informal and formal settings. Beatrix and Thomas describe how they accidentally met the birth parents prior to a contact session and then met them formally during the final contact:

We had to attend contact three times a week. It went on for a couple of months; it was hard but we did it. We would get a call at 9am to tell us if it was going ahead. There was one occasion where the social worker was late and the next minute the birth mother and father came walking through the door. We didn't know what to do. It was actually fine, they were nice people; they are not monsters, they just can't cope. We sat down and asked them questions like '*what is his favourite food?*' It was nice; his dad shook our hand and said thank you. We had final contact in December. We went prepared with a list of questions, but the birth mother didn't want us there, it was too upsetting for her. We gave her a card with their handprints in it.
(Beatrix and Thomas, Foster to Adopt, S five days old, K 22 months, siblings)

3 November

Today we planned to have a quiet day. We have been in such a whirlwind over the last few weeks, with finishing work, the court decision, transition and Jake moving into our home.

This afternoon we geared ourselves up for tomorrow morning – Jake has his final contact session with his birth mother. I am already feeling anxious about it. I have spoken to the social worker and the plan is for a contact social worker to collect him at 10am from our house, then she will bring him back here at 1pm. The journey will be an hour each way and he will be in the contact session for an hour. This will be a long round trip for him. We really have got everything crossed that she attends the session. For Jake and his birth mother, we really want this to happen.

4 November

Today was always going to be difficult. I didn't sleep well last night and woke early worrying about how today would go. Yesterday evening I laid out his clothes, choosing an outfit for him to wear – the final meeting between a birth mother and her child. We chose new clothes, clothes that would only be worn for this meeting and afterwards would be placed in his memory box. I hope this will be a comfort to him one day, knowing that the outfit in the box is what he wore when he was last held and touched by his birth mother.

We were ready early, his bag was packed and we were playing in the living room. I suddenly panicked, I worried that there may be some identifying information in the baby bag, perhaps our names, or our address. I then checked the bag over and over, before being 100 per cent certain that it was fine. I also triple checked that I had packed everything – spare clothes, a bottle, nappies, wipes, toys and a blanket. I also wrote down the timings of his feeds and nappy changes. All I wanted was for Jake to be happy, not to be hungry or upset. I really hoped that this would be well received at the other end.

Then came my second panic. Who was collecting Jake? All we had been told was that he was going to be collected at 10am, no information about who was collecting him. What if we handed him over to an unauthorised person and he went missing? This fear was a little on the irrational side but I couldn't get the thought out of my head. I messaged and rang both of our social workers but there was no answer. It was getting closer to 10am and soon the person would be ringing the doorbell. No response. We had to go ahead. A lady arrived soon after 10am. We made a note of her registration number and the name on her lanyard and handed him over. She said she would be back just after 2pm.

We said goodbye and closed the door. I hugged Will and cried. I was overwhelmed by the enormity and sadness of what was about to happen for Little J. Soon he would be hugged by his birth mother for the very last time; my heart ached for him, for us and for her.

While Jake was away we had set ourselves a series of jobs that needed doing, but as we sat with a cup of tea, we both fell asleep. We were exhausted. We feel as though we are in survival mode at the moment; this is intense.

The social worker and Jake returned just after 2pm, as promised. She came in for a few minutes and told us that all went well; she handed over some gifts from his birth mother, for us to put in his memory box. I am so pleased that the session went as well as could be expected. We have written a few notes from our chat with the social worker; we will share this with him when he is old enough to understand. Unfortunately, because of the timings he missed both of his sleeps for the day. This afternoon we have already seen the knock-on impact; he is very tired and unsettled.

Today has been another emotional day.

5 November

This morning we registered Jake at our local GP practice. In between his feed and his nap we put him in his pram and ceremoniously wheeled him down the road to the doctor. We were proud; this was special. We completed the paperwork and made it clear to the receptionist that they must not, under any circumstances, use his full name when calling him in to see the doctor; this was noted on the system.

On the way home we popped into our local toddler group. I am so glad that Will and I got to do this together for the first time. I was nervous about going into a room of parents with their babies and toddlers – would they know? Could they tell that I didn't know what I was doing? What if he cried and we couldn't settle him? I was feeling the nerves of being a new parent, but with added weight of expectation that really I should know what I am doing with a six-month-old baby.

I need not have been worried, everyone was so lovely. A third of the parents in the room already knew that we had recently been placed with Jake; they were congratulatory and very kind. We sat and chatted while Little Jake lay on the floor with the other babies. It was magical. At the end of the session everyone was invited to the mat for a sing-along. I sat, cross-legged with Little J on my knee. I silently shed a tear. We have waited so long for this moment, to be sitting with a baby, in a toddler group. I glanced at Will and smiled; it was quite overwhelming.

This afternoon our social workers visited. This was the formal handover between our original social worker and the new one. Fortunately they are close colleagues and have a good working relationship; this made for an easy handover. We are so grateful that our original social worker got us through the transition phase. We also had good vibes from our new social worker. I am sure we are going to get on well. Jake was a little unsettled while they were visiting which was a bit of a shame; he has bright red cheeks, he must have a tooth coming through. The pressure when the social workers visit is something that I never really anticipated; we want everything to be just right.

We were given a rough timeline of what happens next. After Christmas we are expected to go to the Matching Panel, then if all goes well, the ADM will approve our placement, then soon after our Fostering for Adoption placement will turn into an Adoption Placement. There is some confusion about when we can apply to the court for the Adoption Order. It is our understanding that the child has to be in your care for ten weeks before making the application. However, there is lack of clarity as to whether this is from the start of the Fostering for Adoption placement, or from when we begin our Adoption Placement.

I have to say, much of what we have been told today has passed over us in a bit of a blur. It all seems so complicated and the social workers have a tendency to talk in acronyms. From our perspective we need to have an overview of the bigger picture, to let us know what we are aiming for, but we also need to focus on the next thing, the next meeting, the next hurdle.

We also spoke about our anxieties of caring for Little J. Will, as ever, is much more relaxed than I am, but given that I am classed as the primary carer, I am really feeling the pressure. I can't help but think about the scenarios that were presented to us during the training – the cases where Fostering for Adoption carers were accused of hurting or harming the child. Every time there is a slight scratch on Jake, I am scared. I think this is also compounded by our experience of being with Jane and David last week. One of the children had cut their hand, and the following day they went for a contact session with their birth mother – a series of allegations followed, against the foster carers. We spoke about these scenarios with our social workers this afternoon. They reassured us that they know the difference between fingernail scratches, accidents and abuse. I desperately want to enjoy this time but living under a cloud of paranoia is very unsettling.

A further aspect of Fostering for Adoption which is difficult to navigate is the language to describe the role you are taking on. We hadn't thought about this prior to placement but soon realised it is a bit of a minefield when you are interacting with the wider professional team which surround this baby. I was constantly scared of saying the 'wrong' thing. All of our family and friends knew that this was a foster placement to begin with but nonetheless the congratulations cards were dropping through our door on a daily basis. I had heard that other Fostering for Adoption carers had been told to take down their cards during formal LAC Reviews, so wasn't sure what the protocol was and what we should do. Looking back, I spent a disproportionate amount of time worrying about this. Beatrix and Thomas describe their experience of this uncertainty and explain how they were told that the cards should come down:

> From day one it felt like we were regarded as babysitters; you have a job as a foster carer, you are not yet a parent. We were told by our social worker at the beginning to 'be Beatrix and Thomas, not mummy and daddy'. This is so hard when you open your hearts to them from the very start. We had congratulations cards from friends and family in the living room; our social worker told us that we should take them down before the guardian came for a meeting.
> (Beatrix and Thomas, Foster to Adopt, S five days old, K 22 months, siblings)

6 November

We had a long and disrupted night with Jake. We are finding that it is a cycle of dummy in, dummy out, dummy in. We don't feel the time is right to take it away from him; this is his constant, his comforter, his safety net.

Mid-morning after his nap we decided to go shopping. It felt like we were preparing for a mission to the moon, but all went well, no dramas. Late afternoon his social worker visited to check all was going well. He was happy and content all afternoon which was lovely for her to see. We asked her permission for an overnight stay. As Will's dad is poorly we have been given permission to stay at their house for two nights this weekend. We are so grateful that the social workers have allowed us to do this. Usually they don't permit any overnight stays within three months of placement, never mind within the first week. Of course we wouldn't have asked if we didn't think it was necessary.

8 November

This morning we were busy, preparing for our first overnight stay. It is unbelievable how many bags we have for a two-night stay. Our life really was so simple before. We have packed his bedding so that it smells of home as well as the monitor – he settles to the sound of his familiar music and likes to see the stars projected on the ceiling. We needed to take two cars with us and I was driving with Jake; the first time driving solo with him. I had a scare en route. He was crying, ear-piercing crying. Then, all of a sudden he stopped. *'Surely babies don't just suddenly stop crying'* I thought. I was panicking, but then saw his hand move – he was okay, he was just asleep. I felt drained by the time I got to Will's parents.

We spent the afternoon doing his usual routine to make him feel settled. He went to bed like a dream, I am so proud of him.

9 November

We had a brilliant night. Jake slept through until 5:40am and he hardly stirred during the night. In the morning, Nanny and I took Jake to a nearly new sale. I have always wanted to go to one of these – we picked up a few bargains. We gave him his bottle while we were there and he was happy in his pram as we walked around the stalls. We did have one awkward moment. One of the stalls had a sling for sale, one of the soft snuggly ones. As I picked it up, looking at the instructions on the box, I was asked how much my little one weighs. My heart dropped. I had absolutely no idea. Out of my mouth came *'I don't know.'* I couldn't even guess, I didn't even know what units baby weights are measured in. Quickly I had to backtrack and justify my lack of knowledge, 'We are adopting him,' I said, 'we have only had him a few days.' Mortified, I quickly paid, and gulped back the lump in my throat.

We timed his afternoon nap for the journey home which worked well. It was so lovely to be able to do this overnight stay, particularly as Grandad has been so poorly in hospital. We are feeling very grateful that it went smoothly, and Jake was so settled.

10 November

Our day started early; he woke at 4am as his nappy had leaked. After a feed in the early hours he went back to sleep for another hour or so. Another first today, we took Jake to the pub in our village for lunch. We met our friends; it was brilliant. Jake had his lunch in the high chair and then went to sleep in the pram – we are calling it beginner's luck. It felt so normal to be out with our baby and friends.

Our cat also seems to have settled into a new routine. Before Jake arrived, if a child came to our house he would run a mile, making a quick exit out of the cat flap. From Day 1 of Little J being in our home, he has stuck around; it is as if he knows that he is here to stay. It looks like these two are going to be best of friends.

11 November

We are coming to the end of Will's parental leave; I am so sad. Unfortunately our transition week is counted as his first week of parental leave, so we have only had one week together at home.

We decided to have a day out together at a local farm park. However, it didn't quite go to plan. When we arrived we realised we had a flat tyre, and the wheel nuts had seized. A phone call to our breakdown cover was needed. We were impressed; they made our call a priority as we were travelling with a baby. We managed to see some of the animals while we waited and had a quick lunch in the café before heading into town to sort out the car. Not quite the relaxing day we had planned, but I am just glad it didn't happen when I was on my own with Jake.

Tomorrow Will goes back to work. The past two weeks have been amazing. We are getting to know Jake's routines, quirks, likes and dislikes. Tomorrow is the start of our new normal. Little J will soon learn that I like to be organised, although I have a feeling he is planning on mixing that up a little bit.

12 November

Last night was my first night of looking after Jake on my own as Will had to be up early for work. He was soaking wet again at 3:30am. He needed a complete change, as well as the bedding. I have no idea what we are doing wrong; the foster carer didn't say that this was a problem. Next time I go shopping I am going to try another brand of nappies.

Mid-morning Jake and I went to our local playgroup. One activity per day is enough for us at the moment. I don't know how people with young children do more than this. I am sure my confidence will grow with time. He was very tired by the time we got home, both of us were very much ready for an afternoon nap.

14 November

Today two amazing friends made a three-hour journey to see Jake and I. They brought a delicious lunch and came prepared with their sleeves rolled up, ready to get stuck in. It was just what I needed on day two of going solo. Over lunch the three of us had a mild panic. Jake had developed a rash around his mouth. The three of us were googling 'baby ... rash ... mouth ... tomatoes' – until we soon realised he had been stabbing himself with a breadstick. They were set to leave mid-afternoon but they insisted on cooking Will and I dinner before making the journey back home. What wonderful friends.

16 November

Today was a special day. We had the first of our very close friends visiting to meet Jake. They have supported us through this journey from day one and were one of our referees. It was so lovely and quite emotional – there were tears. Tomorrow my best friend, her husband and little boy are visiting. She has been another rock throughout this process, and they have shown so much love to Jake. I am so looking forward to our boys growing up together.

19 November

We had a good night. Jake only stirred once at 12:30am. Once again another wet nappy and babygrow; fortunately he didn't wake while we changed him. This morning I went to Rhyme Time at our local library, meeting a friend before the session for a coffee. Jake loved the music and smiled the whole time. After lunch we had our social worker visit. We had a good meeting and talked through Jake's routine and care. We spoke about his habits before he has his milk, crying dramatically before being given his bottle. From the reports we have heard from the foster carers and social workers, we are sure this is a residual impact of trauma from his early days.

We also spoke about the ongoing issue we are having with his nappies. Most nights he is waking up soaking wet. We have now tried every brand of nappy going; you name them, we have tried it.

21 November

We have cracked it – the nappy problem. Last night I was standing watching Will get Jake ready for bed. I watched as he carefully and delicately put on his nappy. Let's just say, it needed to be a lot tighter than that. Source of the problem found – Daddy. However, despite the revelation we didn't have a very good night. He wasn't wet but he was unsettled. We ended up giving him another bottle at 2:30am which did the trick. This morning Little J and I did some jobs around the house and then had our first health visitor check in the afternoon. She had arranged to visit at lunchtime. Before she arrived I was thinking about what to do when she rings the bell. Jake was due to be in his highchair, and I didn't think leaving him in it unattended would be a good idea. I ended up leaving a note on the front door to ask her to let herself in. I thought this was the safest and most appropriate thing to do. I was probably overthinking the scenario once again.

This was the first time she has met Jake. He was an absolute star and she was very complimentary about his development. He is on the 97th percentile for height, which probably means by the time he is about four he will be taller than me. It was also good to know that he is on the 50th percentile for weight – we seem to be feeding him both enough and not too much. She will be attending our Looked After Child Reviews (LAC Reviews) and providing reports to the social workers on his development. We got on really well and it was lovely to get the reassurance that I needed.

24 November

Another unsettled night. This time Will and I were under the covers on our phone googling 'how to get a six-month-old to sleep at 3am.' The top suggestion was 'white noise' to soothe your baby – within minutes it had worked.

Today we drove to my parents' house; we had arranged for my granny to be there to meet Jake for the first time. It was so special, she loved him. He sat on her knee and she took it all in.

29 November

I had arranged to do some Christmas shopping today with Will's parents. Disaster is an understatement. The three of us were in a department store and I said that I would go and change Jake. This was my first time changing him, on my own, in a public place. There was the most cataclysmic explosion I have ever seen and certainly our worst yet. A complete change of clothes was needed – even down to his socks. Then came the 'mummy fail': I had forgotten to pack a spare pair.

I was tired, hot, on my own and I needed a second pair of hands. The tears started to roll, I couldn't believe he didn't have any socks to wear; it was November, he would be freezing. Typically, there was no phone signal in the toilets so I couldn't get hold of nanny. Once we found each other again we sorted the situation by buying him another pack of socks, followed by a cup of tea and a piece of cake; just what I needed. I think we were a bit optimistic doing Christmas shopping trip with a baby in tow this soon into motherhood.

4 December

I had arranged to visit my colleagues at work today. I did the rounds of all the offices with Little J and then had a lovely lunch with a smaller group. He was very much on form and took it all in his stride. Mid-afternoon my throat began to hurt. I thought it was because of all the talking, but by late afternoon I was feeling drained and had a very sore throat and ears.

9 December

All weekend my throat was like a razor blade. Jake was also unwell with a chesty cough and very unsettled during the night. First thing this morning I rang the doctor and booked a double appointment, one for me and one for Jake. He took one look in my mouth and diagnosed tonsillitis for which he has given me antibiotics. He then moved on to Jake. After listening to his chest with a stethoscope, he reassured me that to the naked ear his breathing sounds were worse than it actually is (explaining that this is really common in small children and is usually caused by congestion in the nose and throat). His chest was clear and he said that he should be fine and we should just continue to monitor him.

When we were called in to see the doctor, he used Jake's full name (including his birth surname that remains with him until the Adoption Order is granted). This was despite the safeguarding conversation we had when we registered him. I quickly glanced around the waiting room and fortunately didn't know anyone. After our consultation, I asked the doctor about their safeguarding procedure. He explained that a message comes up on his screen prior to the appointment. When he looked into it, it seemed that an email was covering the safeguarding message. To me, this is an obvious technical flaw. He reassured me that it would not happen again.

11 December

This morning Jake seemed a lot better so I decided to take him to the toddler group. It was a special one; Santa was visiting. During the morning I noticed that one of Jake's fingernails was getting progressively red. One of my friends in the group is a GP. She said that I should call the doctor and get him seen – he has an infection beside his fingernail. I was impressed: I made the call at 11am and by 12:20pm we had an appointment with the doctor – our second within two days. We went straight from the playgroup, with Jake dressed as an elf. It was a good call. The doctor said that he has an infection beside his fingernail and has prescribed a course of antibiotics.

You wouldn't believe it, for the second time this week Jake's name was called out in full by the doctor. This time I was livid (internally), not only because I had already now spoken to them about this twice, but this time I also knew someone in the waiting room. This is so unprofessional and concerning; I am trying to protect the identity of the little one in my care. A formal letter will be sent to the surgery to make a complaint and ask them to review their procedures.

This afternoon we had a social worker visit and she was pleased to hear we had taken Jake to the doctors. She is so pleased with how we are getting on and how we have bonded as a family. We get on really well with her; you can tell that she has a soft spot for Jake. We also discussed our plans for Christmas and we asked her permission to go away for a few nights over the New Year. She said this shouldn't be a problem, we just need to log the addresses and dates that we will be away. She also gave us an emergency number to call, in case we need it over the holiday period.

12 December

As the doctor expected would happen, the infection was much worse this morning. I had been told to relieve the pressure with a sterilised needle, but if I couldn't do it, I should bring him into the surgery. I didn't want to hurt Jake and for him to associate pain with me. My neighbour offered to do it for me. Little J was absolutely fine and hardly flinched. Never a dull moment.

15 December

We met Jane, David, their children and foster children in a lovely café for lunch, halfway between our homes. It was lovely to see them. It seems so long since we were only introducing ourselves and Jake was transitioning into our life – but really it is just over a month. Today it made me realise how much more confident Will and I are. We have really grown to know his little signs, showing us that he is tired or hungry. Their girls loved giving him cuddles and fussing over him. We exchanged cards and presents before heading our separate ways. When Jake arrived, we were messaging them almost daily; now it is weekly. We have said that we would meet up a couple of times a year. We really want Jake to grow up knowing them. They are such an important part of his story.

20 December

This morning Jake's CPR landed on our doorstep. This is the first paperwork we have received since he arrived with us – everything to this point has been verbal. We had just sat down to a lovely breakfast, with music on in the background and Jake playing happily. We decided not to open it – we wanted to enjoy our time together, his first Christmas, and not get stressed or anxious about the details of his case. Our social workers would also be on leave; there was no harm in leaving it until the New Year.

24 December

Christmas Eve is one of my favourite days. We have our own family rituals of finishing the wrapping, having a lovely lunch together and then heading to the crib service at church late afternoon. This was a very special Christmas, his first and our first with him. He loved looking at the lights and listening to the music. When directed, I took Jake up to the nativity scene and we placed a sheep next to the manger – I shed a tear, we had wished for this for so many years.

25 December

Our first Christmas together, what an absolute dream. My parents are staying at our house; it was so lovely to wake up on Christmas morning all together. Jake joined us in bed with his stocking. He had no idea what was going on and he was much more interested in the paper than the presents. This morning we went to our village church, it was so special. As I sat there with J on my lap. I held him tight and smiled thinking back to the 'church alarm incident' – this was a special place for us. Will's parents joined us for lunch and together we celebrated Jake's first Christmas and his first with our family. After lunch, we opened more presents and soon followed a discussion of where on earth we were going to put all of these toys. The one toy basket we began with isn't going to be enough – some major toy storage is needed going forward.

To top the day off, late afternoon our Little J crawled for the first time. So special.

31 December

We had a wonderful few days, going on walks, meeting with friends and relaxing together. This afternoon some family friends visited for tea. They are expecting their own baby soon so it was nice to be able to share some baby tips.

Tonight we are going to one of our neighbours for the street New Year's Eve get together. This afternoon we set up the travel cot in their spare room; we will take him in his pyjamas and put him to bed, then at the end of the evening we will wrap him up and walk the short journey back home and keep our fingers crossed that he transitions back into his cot. Just before we leave to raise a glass to the New Year, Will and I spend some time reflecting on this year.

We began the year filled with hope and expectation. In January, we had just got through the first stage of the adoption process and were about to start Stage 2, the in-depth interviews. Despite the training courses, the books we have read, the advice received, nothing could have prepared us for the rollercoaster we rode this year. In May, we were approved as adopters and then we had five months of waiting and massive decisions before our number 8, our match. Despite the waiting, the let-down, the emotional toil, we are firm believers that 'things happen for a reason'. For us, our reason was Little J. He has now been with us for nearly nine weeks – in fact, 61 days – of family time, giggles, cuddles, crawling and more. Who knows what is in store for the three of us next year, but we hope dearly that we are meant to be together, that this is meant to be.

CHAPTER 8

RETELLING OUR STORY AS A FAMILY OF THREE: PREPARING FOR THE MATCHING PANEL

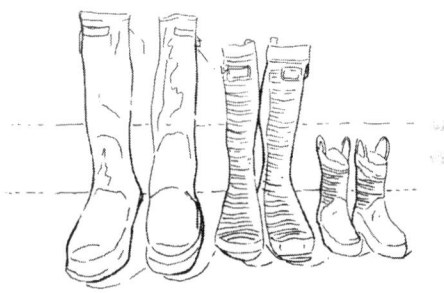

We begin a New Year filled with hope that our family of three will become official. This chapter focuses on the lead up to the Matching Panel and the drama which unravelled as we sat in front of a panel of professionals. It was tense, unsettling, upsetting and above all added another layer of uncertainty – something we weren't prepared for.

2020

1 January

Every New Year's Day our whole street goes for a walk together and end up in the village pub for lunch. It is such a lovely way to start the New Year. We were up early and decided that while Jake had his morning nap we would start reading his CPR – all 48 pages of it. We sat together at the kitchen table and read, line by line, the details of his case. As we went through the document, we made edits and wrote questions in the margin. Midway through we turned the page and saw a photograph of his birth parents; we didn't realise there were going to be photographs included. It upset me; it was the shock more than anything. From the photographs you can quite clearly see that Little J is their baby, the resemblance of features are there. These photographs will be in his life story book; he will grow up with them. When he sees these photographs, he is going to know exactly where he comes from. There will be no ambiguity; he is most certainly their birth child. We hope that this gives him comfort as he grows up.

From reading the document, the statements from multiple professionals and the scenarios that led to Jake entering the care system, it is clear that this was a baby that needed safety and stability. The report revealed without a doubt that a plan for adoption was in his best interest. What was also clear, from reading his report, was that plans for adoption do not stem from one person's perspective; an extensive range of professionals are involved in documenting evidence and providing support to the family. Ultimately, it is the judge who makes the decision after being presented with the evidence. Reading the report this morning reminded me that I needed to hear this; I needed to be sure that we weren't being complicit in a baby not being able to stay with his birth family. I needed to know that adoption was the last resort for Little J and we would do what we could to support him on the next stage of his journey. As we came to the end of the report we had an overwhelming sense of duty, care and responsibility for this little baby in our care. He was with us, and our lives were meant to converge.

Late morning once Jake had woken, we wrapped him up and joined the walk. It was a beautiful, crisp day. Jake was a little star, he loved seeing the other children. Before we sat down to eat, he drank his bottle and then fell fast asleep in the pram for a few hours while we had our lunch. A perfect New Year's Day.

2 January

This morning we carried on looking through the CPR. Alongside providing edits and comments, we were also asked to give answers to a series of questions in anticipation of the panel. One of the questions asked us '*Why do you believe you can provide an adoptive home for this child?*' It seemed that the questions were more suited for a traditional route to adoption, rather than Fostering for Adoption, where the baby had already been placed in our care. This is how we answered:

> We truly believe that this Fostering for Adoption placement was meant to be. Jake has thrived in our care and many developmental milestones are being met. We have an incredible network of friends and family – they all know Jake has been placed with us on an F2A placement; despite this they have showered him with love from day one. Jake is the missing piece to our family and we are excited about what the future holds for the three of us.

Questions answered, paperwork complete, we spent the rest of the morning packing. Before Christmas we decided that it would be nice to go away for a few days in the New Year. The social workers had given us permission for a two-night stay in a cottage. We drove there this afternoon while Jake napped in the car. The cottage is perfect for the three of us, so special to be coming away together, our first trip as a family of three.

7 January

Will was back at work today after the Christmas holiday. I think it is going to take Jake and me a few days to get back into our routine of just the two of us at home in the day. We had a planned social worker visit this morning. She arrived at 9:30am, so we could have a chat before Jake woke from his morning nap. It is a requirement that she sees him awake and interacting. If the social workers visit while he is sleeping, they still have to check him, for safeguarding reasons. We talked through his developmental milestones. He is now sitting, crawling and wanting to stand; he has strong little legs. He is so happy, content and doing well.

We also talked about what happens at the Matching Panel meeting. She told us that there shouldn't be anything to worry about. As we have had Jake in our care, we can easily demonstrate how we have met his needs. Similar to our Adoption Panel, we will be asked questions on our suitability to be parents. I wondered what would happen to Jake while we were in the meeting. At the moment, we are the only people who can look after him and we have already been told that children are not permitted to attend the meeting. She said we would need permission for him to be looked after by my parents. We thought they could go to a café near to the council offices and wait for us.

We were also told about the process post-panel in applying for the Adoption Order. We will need to download an A58 form from the government website. This will need to be completed and submitted with multiple copies of his birth certificate, the Placement Order, our passports, driving licences and marriage certificate. Once we are on the other side of the panel, we will know how many weeks we have to wait before submitting our application (depending on when they count the ten weeks from). It seems strange that this part of the process isn't universal (ie the ten weeks begin at the point of placement). She is optimistic that we may be granted our Adoption Order by May – fingers crossed we have a smooth ride from here.

This afternoon we received our Adoption Placement Report (APR), the document that goes to the panel for matching; this evening we went through it, provided some comments and signed the paperwork for the agency – we are ready for our Matching Panel.

By reading the case studies in the book, hopefully, you will have got the sense that none of this is easy; there is not a one size fits all approach to Fostering for Adoption. Some babies placed on Fostering for Adoption have their Placement Orders, others are still going through court proceedings and the possibilities for family situations and contact arrangements are endless. Some have no contact or just final contact, whereas others have contact multiple times a week for months on end. Charlotte and Richard were desperate for a sibling placement. When they heard about a little boy with a baby sibling on the way, this was their dream, their perfect match. In the case study below they explain how complicated this became with the legal requirements.

> Our hope through the adoption process was to adopt siblings; we also dreamt that we could experience raising a child from birth within a sibling placement. Big Brother had completed his proceedings and had a Care and Placement Order – the plan for him was adoption, via the traditional route. He had a baby sibling on the way that the Local Authority believed they would need to remove at birth. The social workers were looking for a family who had been approved for both adoption and Fostering for Adoption of a sibling group.
>
> Before accepting the match we understood the numerous risks involved. We were fully aware that the various rulings available to the

family court other than an Interim Care Order would result in baby not being placed with us. These included: a Mother and Baby Unit, permanent reunification of baby with biological mother or other extended family member, or reemergence of an as yet unknown biological father.

We also faced the uncertainty regarding the baby's health; baby wasn't born yet and he was small, would he arrive safely? Would he be born prematurely? Would he have any medical conditions that we wouldn't be able to cope with? Ultimately there are no guarantees with the traditional route of adoption but particularly with Fostering for Adoption. The court did grant an Interim Care Order for Little Brother and he was placed in our care from a few days old.

Due to our unique circumstances, and urgency in providing as much time as possible for us all to settle before his baby sibling arrived, the Local Authority initially placed Big Brother as a Fostering for Adoption placement. Within two weeks the Local Authority had completed the linking meeting, foster carer meeting, medical adviser meeting, ADM and all necessary paperwork, as well as placed him in our foster care. We were quickly matched and became an Adoptive Placement soon after.

We then thought that after ten weeks of placement we would be able to apply for an Adoption Order for Big Brother. Unfortunately, we were informed that if an Adoption Order was granted for Big Brother we would no longer be classed as approved adopters and would need to be re-approved to adopt Little Brother. Our agency advised against this, therefore we delayed submitting an Adoption Order application for Big Brother until Little Brother had gone through his court proceedings.

Considering our circumstances we believed this was the correct decision for us; it would have been too much to go through the approval process at the same time as caring for both of the boys and all of what the Fostering for Adoption process entailed.

If the court had decided reunification with birth family was possible for Little Brother, birth family could have then contested the Care and

Placement Orders granted for Big Brother as he was only placed for adoption, not yet legally adopted. The risks we were taking felt so much greater because we went into our link believing that we would be able to adopt Big Brother no question, and thought the uncertainties were only with Little Brother.

Throughout the process we felt like we had no power. It's very difficult when you become parents and take them in as though they have always been yours but knowing that you have no parental responsibility and they could be picked up tomorrow and you would have no legal claim to them.

We coped with this by living in the present – trying to not let the fear and uncertainty of the process steal away the joy of each day spent with these boys. To trust in the process and want whatever outcome was best for them, not best for us; to become parents and put their needs before our own.

(Charlotte and Richard, Foster to Adopt, siblings, weeks apart, one from foster care and a baby from hospital)

14 January

Jake and I made the two-hour journey to see one of my old school friends. We only see each other every few years, but when we do it is like the good old days. She also has a little one and is on maternity leave, so we thought it would be lovely to meet up. Last weekend I found some toy storage advertised online; it just so happened that the address for the collection was near to where she lives. Everything went to plan. We met for a cup of tea in the morning, then I collected the storage unit. Rather than heading straight home, I decided to have lunch in town with Jake.

While in the café my phone rang. It was Jake's social worker, her name flashed up on my phone. My heart skipped a beat; it always does when she calls. What has happened? What was wrong? She was ringing to tell me that, unfortunately, she won't be able to attend our Matching Panel next week, as she has booked her annual leave. The plan is for her line manager to attend on her behalf. Obviously, I understand that social workers also need to have holidays and they will always be missing something, but as we have got on so well it would have been calming to have her there. She reassured us that her manager knows the case as well as she does and we don't have anything to worry about. The news could have been worse; at least the panel is still going ahead next week.

21 January

Tomorrow is our Matching Panel, another big day. I have to say though we are feeling quite relaxed about it. We have been caring for him for the past few months and are completely head over heels in love with him – I am sure this will come across as we speak. My parents are going to meet us in the council car park beforehand; they will then take Jake to a café and give him his bottle while we are in the panel meeting. Fingers crossed all goes smoothly.

22 January

Panel day. We were in a rush this morning, getting Jake ready and trying to get to the council office with time to spare. What we didn't take into account was the ice on the roads, rush hour traffic and a shortage of car park spaces in the centre of town. After a 30-second handover with my parents, which in turn made them stressed, we called our social worker as we were running to the council offices. We made it with a minute to spare. We are never late for anything, so this of all the days was not ideal.

This was a sign of things to come.

We entered the room flanked by our social worker and the social worker manager that had stepped in last minute. Similar to our Adoption Panel, sat in a horseshoe were the panel members – the Chair, the Secretary, a foster carer, a social worker, the medical adviser and an independent panel member. Unlike before, I wasn't nervous. We entered the room knowing that we knew Jake better than anyone else, and in our hearts we knew that this was the perfect match for us.

After a quick round of introductions, the questions began. This is where it began to unravel in front of us. For confidentiality and Jake's privacy, I can't be specific about the questions or our responses but the first question that we were presented with hit us like a ton of bricks. I think our faces said it all; we had no idea what they were talking about. I managed to provide a generic, brief answer but the reality was that I had no idea what the question was referring to. I looked at Will for reassurance and I could tell he was panicking as well; he didn't have anything to add.

My initial feeling was that Will and I looked unprepared. It came across as though we hadn't read the CPR properly. Whizzing through my head I was thinking about the line-by-line way that Will and I went through the document; how could we have missed such a significant detail about Jake's life? I remember looking at the faces of the panel members and wondering what they were thinking about us. After some confusion and awkwardness then came the second question. We couldn't answer this one either. I looked at Will, again a blank face, I couldn't understand it, we had been over that document with a fine-tooth comb. Then the penny dropped. I was 100 per cent certain, I said '*I don't think we have been reading the same version of the paperwork*.' The panel looked at one another and then the Chair began to flick through the document, asking, did we know this, or that, or had we seen the photographs on page 27? The answer to all of this was, '*no we hadn't*.' After some detective work during the panel, it seemed that the panel had been sent the most recent version of Jake's CPR and we hadn't. The Chair then asked us to leave the room with our social worker and the manager. It was tense. We sat in an adjoining room. We couldn't believe it; how had this happened? The four of us sat and tried to work out what had gone wrong, how had we ended up with the wrong version? However, that part was irrelevant, it had happened. We had a bigger problem. The disclosures that were raised by the panel asking these two questions were significant. In fact, if we had known the full extent of the issue prior to placement, I was sure that this would have been a difficult decision for Will and I to make. However, things were different now, Little J was part of our life and our story. We would of course take him and his full story and all the risks that this entailed. We were committed to him. We talked this through with our social workers while the panel deliberated.

The panel on the other hand had made a decision: they wanted to give us the option to suspend the meeting. They agreed that we shouldn't progress as we have not been given the correct paperwork to be able to make an informed decision about being matched with Jake. We were given time on our own to make a decision as to how to progress. For us, yes, a mistake had been made, but from our perspective, we were committed to Little J – whatever his background and story, he was now part of our story and we wanted to go ahead; no hesitation, both of us agreed.

Once we were ready, we were ushered back to the panel meeting. We made our feelings known and the panel agreed that (a) we wanted to proceed; (b) we would be sent the correct version of the paperwork; and (c) we would confirm our position in writing.

Before we left, the panel were keen to have a conversation about our thoughts on meeting Jake's birth mother. We were told that she has requested to meet us before the adoption goes through; we are grateful of this. We want to be able to tell Jake that we had met her, had an opportunity to ask her questions and hopefully have a photograph together. For him this is really important. We also want her to know that we are going to take care of him, unconditionally.

We also spoke about the importance of maintaining contact with Jane and David. They are an important part of his life; they were there from the beginning. They will be able to answer questions that Will and I as his daddy and mummy will never be able to answer. The panel seemed happy with our reflections and plans moving forward; all in the best interests of Jake.

Before we left the council office, we were handed the 'correct' version of the paperwork to take away with us. Our social worker was devastated about what had unfolded in the meeting; she said it was the worst panel experience she has ever had.

We had been in the meeting for two hours. I quickly rang my parents who were of course worrying. They were convinced something terrible had happened and were expecting the worst – that we hadn't been matched with Jake. Over lunch, we talked through the drama as it had unfolded and reassured them of our intention to continue with our Little J, despite the new risks that this entailed.

23 January

We woke up feeling angry with what had happened yesterday. We went to bed late last night after we had scanned through the two versions of the CPR that we had been given. They were certainly different. There was much more information, including photographs of other family members, in the second version.

While Jake slept, I went through both documents, line-by-line, and made a note of all the inconsistencies. Across the 60 pages, there were 15 sections of the report with either missing or changed information; it took me two hours. Despite this, other than the two major omissions that were mentioned yesterday at the panel, the other details were contextual and not so much of an issue. We emailed our social workers to make it explicitly clear that we wanted to proceed with adopting Jake, but of course, we were disappointed that this had happened. Readers may want to know what the missing information related to. As I say, I can't for confidentiality reasons disclose this but I will give some scenarios to give a sense of the severity. The CPR documents contain information related to: the child's birth parents and siblings; the views of the guardian; a chronology of care since birth; detailed description of the child, social, emotional, physical characteristics; medical; education; family history; and extensive reports from professionals relating to the reasons the child is being adopted (see CoramBAAF, 2018). If any of the sections are missing or incomplete, then the adopters are not going to be fully informed.

From the beginning of the process we have been so organised with the paperwork; you have to be. We have written everything down, every small detail. When we told our family and friends about what happened yesterday, their immediate response was *'you should complain'* – however, it is not as easy as that. During the process we have always felt beholden to the system; we don't want our chances of adopting a child to be jeopardised. Clearly an error was made somewhere along the line, we don't know by whom or how, but we know that mistakes happen and it was just unfortunate that it happened to us. In this case, it is fortunate, particularly for Jake, that we as his adopters want to proceed.

Later on this afternoon, I took Jake for his scheduled health check at our local surgery. They weighed him and they are pleased with how well he is doing. It was suggested that we might want to drop his morning bottle and go straight into breakfast. Just when we thought we had cracked the current routine, there is a change.

25 January

I had a wonderful morning with a friend and her daughter. We had booked a session in a sensory playroom. There were lights, bubbles, toys, beautiful sounds and lots of other sensory materials that Jake loved exploring. When I was 18, I spent time volunteering at a children's hospital and the sensory room was a particular highlight for the children. I came home from our adventure this morning and announced to Will that we needed to make Jake a sensory board – a must-have accessory for any toddler. This will be a weekend project, our first stop will be the shed to see if we have any surplus bolts, door handles and switches.

28 January

It is time for our weekly session of Rhyme Time at our local library. I am impressed as over 80 children and carers attend each week. We all sit on the carpet for 30 minutes of singing and music-making.

This afternoon I had a few calls with the social workers going over the issues which were raised at the panel. I have also been working on my daily logs which I need to hand over to the social workers before our LAC Review. I tend to write bullet point notes on the day on my phone and then once a week spend a few hours typing up the report to send on to the team. I thought it would be useful to share one of my daily log entries (the one below is for today). How they look may vary depending on the requirements of the social worker team and agency, but we were asked to submit our logs in the format shown below – highlighting sleep, food, activities, any medication and amount of milk.

When Jake arrived we downloaded an app to track and log all of his feeds, nappy changes, sleeps and food. Both of us had the app and could update from our own phones. We found this really useful not only for our logbook writing but to get to learn his rhythms, likes and dislikes.

28 January	- Woke at 6:20am
	- Breakfast – cereal and toast
	- This morning we went to the library for Rhyme Time, J loves to play with the musical instruments
	- J had a sleep in the car on the way home
	- Lunch – sweet potato, chicken and harissa seasoning
	- In the afternoon I had a series of calls from the social workers to discuss the issues raised at the panel
	- Play time and stories
	- Dinner – scrambled egg
	- Gave J medicine today for his teeth
	- 11 oz of formula (less than usual)
	- Bed at 7:10pm

5 February

The toddler group in our community is important. Volunteers in the village put so much effort into making it a special place for parents, carers and their little ones. Up until now, I have been able to sit on the baby mat and have a good chat with the other parents while our little ones lie or sit in one place. Not anymore. Today Jake started to explore; he wanted to play with the big toys. He even crawled through one of the tunnels; he definitely has an adventurous streak. He slept well this afternoon after all that playing and stimulation.

Tomorrow we have got our Looked After Child meeting, also known as an LAC Review. These happen at set times throughout the process, led by the IRO and attended by all professionals who are involved in the care of the child. Our social worker rang this afternoon to check if I was happy with the format. She knows that I will have my hands full with Jake and showing everyone into the house, so she has offered to make everyone tea and coffee. I have said I will leave everything out to make it easy for her.

Will will be at work tomorrow, so I am feeling anxious about doing this on my own. It is hard not to think that all eyes are going to be on me – with everyone in our living room thinking, how is she coping? Has Jake attached? Is he safe, happy and well? I have just got to keep calm and take this one for the team. I am sure it will be fine.

6 February

Our LAC Review was scheduled for 10am this morning. As expected I woke up early feeling nervous. I had planned the whole morning. I would put him down for his nap a bit early, so that he may then wake at 9:45am, which would give me 15 minutes to get him up, dressed and presentable before the team arrive. Before he was up in the morning and after Will went to work I ran around the house, tidying up the shoes, making the kitchen shine, tidying away any stray toys and finally getting out the cups ready for the tea to be made. Short of getting Jake ready, I was ready.

At 9:46am my phone rang. It was Jake's social worker; she had just received a call from the IRO that he was sick and so would not be able to attend. I couldn't believe the meeting had been cancelled at this late notice. Our other social worker and the health visitor would be well on their way; she had to phone them quickly as well.

I was exhausted. So much emotion goes into preparing for a meeting like this; to be let down at the last minute is so frustrating. With a free morning now ahead of us, Jake and I went into our nearest town and scouted the charity shops for some bits and pieces for his sensory board.

10 February

A day of two extremes. This morning I was out for a lovely walk with Jake; he was in the pushchair and I was singing to him. My phone rang. As I took it out of my pocket I could see Jake's social worker was calling. *'What now?'* I thought.

She sounded in a panic. She said *'Alice, I have had to sit down to read the email in front of me.'*

I had no idea what she was talking about, or what she was about to say, but I felt sick.

'It says that you and Will don't want to continue with Jake's placement', she continued.

WHAT? I am sure the colour must have drained from my face. I stood there with pram in one hand and phone in the other, and felt like the air had been punched from my stomach.

I didn't find out who the email was from or where on earth they had got that information, but it was incorrect. There was nothing that Will and I have said to any of the professionals involved that would cause them to doubt our love and commitment to Jake. Of course, she knew this and was quick to offer her reassurance that she thought there must have been some misunderstanding along the line of communication. I felt sick because I realised that in one phone call, one email, one misinformation everything can change, just like that. I did what I could to reassure her and asked her to communicate this to the wider team – we are committed to this little boy, full stop.

After this drama, later on in the afternoon, we had an unexpected email from our social worker. She was writing with the great news that today marks the end of our fostering period. We are now officially out of the riskiest phase and going forward there is now no requirement for us to write our daily logs. Looking back, I am pleased that we now have his first few months documented in such detail. Hopefully he will enjoy reading it one day. Tonight I submitted our last documents to the fostering team.

I can't quite believe the rollercoaster of today – from the panic this morning to the relief this afternoon.

For us, our fostering period was relatively short. Some families have to endure months and months of uncertainty. Sam and Alexander had no intention of doing Fostering for Adoption. During their training, they decided they didn't want the risk. Despite this, they ended up accepting a baby on a Fostering for Adoption placement with a planned court date two days later. Plans soon shifted and at the time of writing, they were in a state of anxiety with no Placement Order and with a birth relative being reassessed by the order of the judge. Here they share their story:

> During our training and assessment we had considered Fostering for Adoption but concluded that it was not for us; we didn't want to go

down this risker route. A little boy stole our heart. We saw his profile at a workshop; three months later we went to panel. Once we were approved, he was still available for adoption – a meeting was arranged. The evening before we were due to meet we got a call from our social worker to inform us that the foster carers had decided they wanted to adopt the boy. To say we were gutted is an understatement.

A month later our social worker informed us of a potential match. The case was in court; we were cautious and anxiously awaited information on the outcome. Another month passed and we were informed that if everything goes ahead the little girl would come to live with us within days. We were hopeful and we were told that due to some circumstances we would have the little one living with us on an early placement for two days, as the court date was a couple of days after the placement. We were okay with that – after all it would only be for two days – or so we thought. It has now been two months; as yet, no Placement Order has been granted. We are devastated, we did not want to be in this position – the pain of not feeling prepared for this heartache and feeling alone. The last court date was a few days ago; we are still reeling. A birth relative is being reassessed; even though the previous assessment was negative the judge decided to reassess. If the reassessment is positive we have been told the baby will be moved into a foster home before Christmas as a bridge before the final hearing. This situation is so heartbreaking; we are worrying day and night. My partner has gone back to work but his mind is not fully there – we are having sleepless nights, feeling sick but trying to be hopeful. We are fearing the worst and hoping for the best. We did not want to be in this situation; we did not want to do Fostering for Adoption. Our main priority is the little one; she needs us and as much as we need her. We so much want to call this baby girl our own – she needs us to stay positive but we cry when she is sleeping. This is not what we signed up for, but we are hoping for a happy ending.

(Sam and Alexander, Foster to Adopt, girl, six months)

15 February

I am in Suffolk with Jake and my mum staying with my godmother. Of course, we had to get permission for this trip. Even though we are officially out of the fostering period, our agency still requires us to log where we are going and when. We are so grateful that he is so content and seems to sleep anywhere, as long as we stick to his routine.

Today we took him to the beach. This is his first trip to the seaside; being February it was a little bracing but lovely. In the New Year, Will and I set a challenge: we want to take Jake to every county in England (there are 27 of them) by the time he is five. There are a few rules though: (i) we have to stay overnight in the county, passing through is not allowed; (ii) on each visit we need to buy a postcard and take a photograph; and (iii) we need to write on the back of the postcard to remind us of the visit. Today we managed to find a lovely postcard in Southwold, so were able to stage a beautiful photograph on the beach – this is our fifth county since he arrived.

17 February

We arrived back from Suffolk last night. We needed to be home with Jake because today was our rescheduled LAC Review. It was another busy morning of packing away all the luggage, hoovering and tidying up.

Our review was at 11am, timed for when Jake would be awake from his morning nap. Jake was a super star, I was so proud of him. We spent time talking through the issues that were raised in our panel meeting, our Adoption Order paperwork, the life story books, the Later Life letter, Letterbox contact and developmental milestones. The IRO was lovely; he was really reassuring, confident and calm. He explained that he had been involved in Jake's case from Day 1. He spoke from the heart when he said '*I am just so delighted with this placement. This is the best outcome for Jake, his life chances have dramatically changed.*' Of course, I cried. I really felt like he meant it and he was certain that it was in Jake's best interests that adoption was the right plan for him and his future. The team left after nearly two hours. As I closed the door, I hugged Little J and shed a happy tear. They were nothing but complimentary and it was so lovely to hear.

18 February

This morning it was Jake's adoption medical. It is a requirement that Looked After Children under the age of five have a medical assessment every six months. Our appointment was at 10am in another city. We decided that Will's mum would come with me, so that we could both listen to the consultant and she could be there to hold Jake if I needed to write notes. Our assessment went well, and the medical adviser was pleased with his developmental progress.

19 February

Another mini-holiday, another county ticked off our list. We are now in Wiltshire. Before we left, we booked an appointment to see a potential nursery. We have been keen to get his name on a list. I have to say we loved it. I can't imagine a more perfect setting for Little J. It was beautiful; all of the materials they use are natural and they are guided by a curiosity-led approach. At one point, we put Jake on the floor. He crawled to the toys and started playing – it was so lovely to see. After our tour, we had a meeting with the manager. We were able to ask about their understanding of therapeutic parenting and their experience of working with Looked After Children. We were impressed with their understanding. They wanted to know about any potential triggers and attachments. We explained that we felt that he had formed strong attachments to us since moving into his new home. We also spoke about their policy with photographs, both internal and on social media. We made it clear that we wanted his status as an adopted child to be private, but in no way a secret. We want him to grow up knowing that there are all kinds of families and love is what binds them together. We are so happy that we have found a nursery that I am sure Jake will thrive in. It is a two-minute walk from my office too, so that is such a bonus.

We then made the journey to our cottage for the weekend. We stopped on the way for dinner at a pub. The table next to us were full of compliments, saying how gorgeous and well behaved he was – so lovely to hear, another proud parent moment. We arrived at the cottage just in time for his bath. Once in his cot, he was out like a light.

20 February

I don't think we will forget this visit to a farm. Primed with our latest county postcard and a backdrop of the farm animals, I rather dramatically fell into a pile of poo. As it was a community-led farm initiative with a distinct lack of facilities, I had to make do with a hosepipe to clean myself down. There is never a dull moment in the life of Alice, Will and Little J.

24 February

For Christmas our parents bought Jake swimming lessons. Today my mum met me at the pool. We had a quick lunch, then he napped in the pram before the lesson began. He loved it; he splashed, smiled, laughed and was very forthcoming with all the activities. I have always been a water baby; I really hope he grows up loving the water as much as I do.

29 February

Tonight we stayed with my best friend. Her little boy adores Jake; he has told his teachers at school that he has a little brother, so sweet. She has been there through every stage of this process with me, from the assessment to panel, to waiting, matching, introductions, the early days and everything in between. Tonight we asked her and her husband if they would be godparents to Jake. They were delighted to be asked. I know they will be strong role models as he grows up and will be there if he needs them. It was a special evening, one we will remember.

4 March

For the first time since Jake arrived, we were able to leave him with his grandparents for a few hours. I had some work I needed to do, so I went to a nearby café while nanny and grandad looked after him. They said he was settled and played well. We have seen them a lot since Jake came home, so I am sure he feels safe and secure with them. Once I return to work the arrangement will be that he spends a day with each of his grandparents. We are so pleased that he will have this opportunity to build a strong relationship with them, as we did with our grandparents.

7 March

Jake is growing so fast, it was time for a wardrobe upgrade. This time last year we were buying baby items for an unknown little one. It made us feel uneasy and anxious – we were effectively spending money on an unknown gender and age of baby. Now of course we know exactly what we need and what size – it is a wonderful feeling.

10 March

We have been sent a copy of a life story book that has been made for Jake. This is intended to be a child-friendly version of his story. I have to say we are not very happy with it – the language used or the formatting. I replied to his social worker, thanking her for the document. I know that social workers are overworked and have limited resources but more time needs to be allocated to life story work – for the long-term benefit of the children. I have said that I would use this as a template and work on our own version – more child-friendly, more appropriate and with more love woven into the pages.

11 March

This morning we had Jake's health visitor assessment. We entered the room, set up with toys and activities. He crawled around the room looking at the toys, but then would look back at me for reassurance. It was brilliant; this was attachment in practice, I felt so proud. We went through all of his routines including sleep, food and milk and she was very pleased with his progress. He is *'meeting all of his developmental milestones'* – a phrase I am sure is a relief to any parent at one of these assessments. I was beaming from ear to ear when she left. I was given reassurance; as his parents we are doing everything we need to be doing to support him.

12 March

Today, we visited my birth father's tree, a sapling that was planted in his memory that now stands metres tall. This is the first time we have taken Jake so it was a special visit.

I was one when my dad died – I now stand in front of the tree with a one year-old that has come into our lives and hearts.

From great oaks, little acorns grow.

CHAPTER 9

FORMALISING OUR STORY: APPLYING FOR THE ADOPTION ORDER AND EVERYDAY FAMILY LIFE

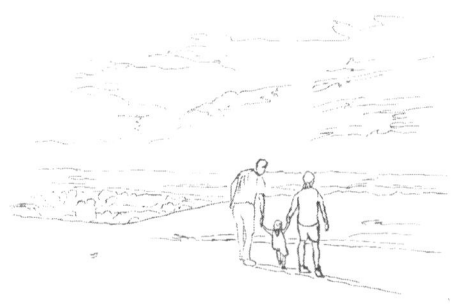

Twenty weeks ago we opened the foster carers' front door, looked down and saw Jake looking up at us. This was the beginning. Officially we have been his carers, reporting to social services everything he has consumed, all that he has done, where he has been and who he has met. Importantly though, we have spent our days learning how to be a mummy and daddy.

There have been moments where we have been seriously tested by the process. There have been tears and lots of worry. Despite this, we have been with Jake as he learnt to sit, crawl, stand, giggle, cuddle and more – these were his firsts, and we feel privileged to have been able to share these with him. We now know him better than anyone.

Over the next few months our Adoption Order paperwork will be submitted to court and the final decision made. This chapter documents the formalising of our story – the final stage of the process.

19 March

Today we posted our adoption application, our formal paperwork to the court. What an amazing feeling, to be another step forward in formalising our family of three. The paperwork wasn't too onerous, but some of the questions were a little ambiguous, so we ran these past our social worker. We also had to get various copies of documents including birth certificates, driving licences, passports, our marriage certificate and the fee payable to the court. When I was writing out the cheque, I was thinking that this was the first payment we have had to make in the whole adoption process. I have spoken to friends in other countries where the fees for adoption can cost thousands of pounds – I am sure this adds a whole other dimension to the process.

Tonight we raised a glass, one step closer to our forever life with Little J.

22 March

Mothering Sunday. My first as a mummy. On Mothering Sundays in the past, I have thought about my mummy and her mummy, close friends of mine whose mummies are no longer with us and those who are desperate to be a mummy. This year I add to this list; today especially I am thinking about a mummy whose little one I am currently caring for with all the love I have to give. This little one binds us both together – two people, two mummies, who have not met but have one thing in common, our Little J. This year I am on my way to becoming Jake's forever mummy, and for this, I feel truly blessed.

I was recently asked how soon I knew that I was in love with him. For me this is easy to answer. I knew how much I loved him after a week of him being in our care – the day he went for his final contact session with his birth mother. On this day I knew it, I knew that I loved him. I wanted this last moment with his birth mother to be special. I dressed him in a new outfit, he was gorgeous. I wanted this to be special for them both. Another way I knew that love was blossoming was due to the anxiety I felt about him leaving us for a few hours. I wanted him to be okay, to be safe.

A few months earlier, I had a similar question. *'How much do you love him?'* they asked.

'My love exceeds every metaphor going,' I replied.

I would put my life in front of his if I needed to – this is how I know I am in love.

23 March

Tonight there was a ministerial broadcast. Boris Johnson announced that the UK will be going into a national lockdown to curb the spread of Covid-19, a virus that is spreading globally. There will be no mixing with other people, only one form of exercise is allowed each day and you can only leave the house if you are a key worker, for food supplies or to access health care.

There has been speculation that this may happen for a few weeks; but now, as the official announcement has been made there is shock and panic among our family, friends and the wider population.

25 March

We are now a few days into social distancing, and I am feeling really down. Like everyone, I can't believe this has happened and we are all facing these restrictions. Who would have thought my parental leave would have been spent in a national lockdown? No baby groups, no socialising with other parents, no swimming, no parks, and of course the hardest part of all, not seeing our family and friends. We have waited for so many years for these special times and now we can't share them with anyone or go anywhere.

26 March

Today we have had some bad news. Due to Covid, all court proceedings have been put on hold. To be delayed at this stage is so frustrating. In a few days, we were due to hear if his birth parents would be contesting the adoption. Now we are unlikely to know for weeks, if not months. Coupled with lockdown this is really tough. This is going to mean more months of us living in limbo. The thought of not having Jake in our lives is unthinkable. We have to carry on believing that this is the right pathway for him and we are meant to be his parents. I have also been feeling sad for all the babies and children who will now, without a doubt, be stuck in the system for longer, as well as the children that will end up in care as a result of the pandemic.

I imagine that we are all going to feel down at some point during the lockdown. This evening Will and I have had a chat. We need to keep focusing on the positives. We have lots to be positive about – we have a beautiful, happy, content baby asleep upstairs, a baby who we love more than we ever knew was possible.

We have decided that we will video call both of our parents every day, so they can see Jake and he can see them and recognise their voices. Over the last few months, we have worked hard to build a relationship between Jake and his grandparents; it is so important that he continues to recognise them. In the morning while he is having his breakfast, we will video call my parents and then at the end of the day, before bed, speak to Will's. This will also give us a routine and structure to our day which we need. There is another reason to be happy, the three of us are at home together – we will be able to slow down and appreciate all the moments as this little one grows and develops, day by day.

28 March

While Jake has been napping in the day or sleeping at night, we have been working on his life story book. Last night I finished the first draft and shared a copy with our social workers. We have decided to make two versions. The first is aimed at age one to six, then the second, for when he is a little older and begins to ask more questions. Both are written and designed using age-appropriate language and images. During our training, we learnt the importance of life story work and were able to see some examples of books that were produced by social workers and families. Life story work was considered important for the following reasons.

1. It allows the child to make sense of their past and present life so that they can move into the future with confidence.
2. It gives the child a structured and understandable way of talking about themselves.
3. It is a chronology of the child's life.
4. It offers clarity where there are dangerous or idealised fantasies.

5. It increases a child's sense of self-worth and self-esteem.

6. It provides an opportunity to show children why they should be proud of themselves.

7. It is important to tell the truth, however painful.

(Notes adapted from our agency training)

From the examples of life story books we have been shown, there is a preferred order to the information presented: (i) it is most common for the book to begin with the child and their adoptive parents, to show belonging and security; (ii) the book then progresses to address any early trauma and their history with birth family; and (iii) ends by promoting attachment and belonging. Through all of our training, it has been reinforced on many occasions that as adoptive parents it is our 'responsibility to keep our child's story alive'.

By late afternoon, our social workers had replied – they love the book. They even went so far as to say that it should be used as an exemplar within the agency. They appreciate all of the work we have put into it. They have asked us if they can share it among their team, to inspire other social workers as to what is possible in life story work.

14 April

Today, Jake and I put on our outdoor gear and set out for the hills. It was a beautiful day. While we were out on our mini adventure, I thought back to the time when he arrived. For a good few months we were in survival mode. In the early days, I couldn't imagine being confident enough to take him out on my own, never mind putting him in the backpack and heading for the hills with an OS map. We have certainly grown in confidence together. If you are reading this and are yourself currently in survival mode with a new addition to your family, trust me, you will be able to do more than one thing per day – go shopping with a little one in tow and even have mini adventures – just take your time, there is no rush.

18 April

The weather was terrible today, which called for one thing – messy play. I cleared out a large plastic storage box, got out a plastic sheet and set up a messy play station in the kitchen while Jake had his morning nap. I whisked up two tins of chickpea liquid and made a bowl of aquafaba. When he woke, we put him in a nappy and vest and popped him in the plastic box with the toys and foam. At first, he wasn't sure what to make of being swiftly taken from his cot and right into a messy play station, but we soon got smiles and he had a sneaky taste of the foam. To clear down we gave him a bath in the sink. This is what wet and windy mornings are made for.

21 April

Tonight, for the first time, Jake pressed the button on his baby monitor to activate the stars. He craned his head up to the ceiling and smiled. This is his routine – his stars, his music. We will continue to use it for as long as he needs.

The baby monitor was one of the first 'baby items' that we bought after we were approved. We thought this was a safe bet; regardless of age or gender, we were sure we would need a monitor. We spent time researching the various features. Did we need one with a screen? A motion sensor mat for the crib? Long range? The choices were quite overwhelming. We settled on one and we were excited, a step closer to being parents. Little did we know, our baby would come with his own monitor – one which shines stars on the ceiling and plays a rhythmic tune. Every night since birth he has looked up at those stars.

1 May

My first birthday as a mummy. It began with a wonderful 11 hours sleep; Little J timed that well, what a treat. This morning we had our scheduled LAC Review, via video link, of course, because of Covid. I was pleased that Will could also attend as he is working from home and would now meet our IRO. It was a good meeting, attended by us as the adopters, the IRO, Jake's social worker, our social worker and the health visitor. Everyone is very happy with the placement and they were very complimentary towards Will and me. The only disappointing news is that our court date has once again been delayed due to Covid, but of course, this is all out of our control.

After the meeting, we went for a walk in the sunshine and then had a lovely lunch in the garden; it felt like summer and the weather was beautiful. I had a fun afternoon wrapping Jake's birthday presents. I think many of my birthdays, going forward, are going to be spent wrapping his presents, how wonderful. Late afternoon we had a video call with our parents and then we ended the day with a socially distanced drink in the garden through the fence with our next-door neighbours and treated ourselves to a takeaway curry.

10 May

One year ago today, at exactly the same time that Will and I were in our panel meeting, baby Jake was born. If this isn't fate, I don't know what it is.

A lockdown first birthday wasn't ideal. Pre-Covid, we had planned to have a party for him, with the hope that our Adoption Order was through, but sadly this didn't work out. Nevertheless, we planned a special lockdown day for him. Mid-morning we had a video call with our parents and they watched us open presents. Next, we went for a lovely walk in the sunshine, with a balloon of course. Then we set up camp in the garden; we decided that we would try camping with him for the first time – a birthday under canvas. In the late afternoon, we had another video call with all of our friends and family, from neighbours on our street to friends in the USA – everyone joined us with a cup of tea and a piece of cake. We blew out his candles and sang 'Happy Birthday' to him. We are so grateful to all of our friends and family for making his first birthday one to remember; it was so special.

Camping with a one year-old and no experience – let's just say it was a good job we were only in the garden. We did his normal bedtime routine but instead of milk and a story on the sofa, we moved into the tent. We made the decision to use our small tent, thinking it might be warmer. This was a mistake. It took him ages to get to sleep – far too busy crawling around, investigating all the zips and pockets. What we hadn't accounted for was the weekly clap for carers – at 8pm the clapping, claxons and car engines sounded. Not surprisingly, he woke and it wasn't until dark that he finally drifted off again. Will and I had a BBQ and drinks around the firepit, a perfect end to a perfect day. Fingers crossed for a good night under canvas.

11 May

It was a night to remember. All was fine until Jake woke at 2am. Wide awake he was crawling around the tent singing 'row row boat'. We lasted

45 minutes and then decided to go back into the house. By 3am he was back in his cot and fast asleep and didn't wake until 7:30am. Next time we will use the big tent and keep him in the cot.

14 May

Today we had a call from our social worker. We have been asked if we will accept birthday and Christmas cards from Jake's birth mother. This shocked us a bit. In all of the training there was no mention of cards, only the annual Letterbox contact. Of course, we want him to be able to have cards from his birth mother, but we think it needs to be handled sensitively. We are anxious about cards arriving, or not, in the lead up to special occasions and the impact this will have on Jake, and of course us as a family. Our social worker had a good idea; she suggested that once a year, aligned with our allocated month for Letterbox contact, cards can also be sent, for the following Christmas and birthday. We are happy with this suggestion; we are glad we have a solution that is in Jake's best interests.

19 May

This morning, Jake had his one-year immunisation. He is terrified of the visors and personal protective equipment (PPE) that the doctors and nurses wear. We hadn't even got through the door and he was hyperventilating, poor little boy. This Covid world must be so scary for children. I think we are going to have to start playing a game with the masks to get him used to them.

24 May

Before Little J arrived, I don't think I appreciated how important teddies were for attachment. He has four little beauties that snuggle up with him each night. Let me introduce you. We have Lamby, our newest birthday addition to the crew; she is the softest and is purely for bedtime snuggles. Next is Bear, one of our originals; he knows how bedtime works and is always the first to be kissed. Then there is Bunny; he has a soft spot in all our hearts. He has seen it all. As the transition Bunny, he will always be number one. Then lastly Doggo, the most adventurous. He is the one that comes with us on special trips to make sure Jake is doing just fine. We love these teddies, they are part of our family and his routine.

26 May

We had a shock today. Mid-morning we had a call from the 'Letterbox coordinator' – a birthday card had arrived for Jake from his birth mother. We were told that we might find the content upsetting and she wanted to know what she should do with it; she gave us the option of leaving it on his file at the agency. We asked her to send it to us. Due to Covid, there has been mixed and delayed communication and the agreed Letterbox strategy hasn't been implemented this year. She has warned us that we might be upset.

We have also been asked to write a 'Settling in letter'. Many birth parents are anxious about the impact of Covid on their children and need reassurance that they are safe and well. After lunch we sat down and drafted the letter, reassuring her that he is settled, happy and content. We told her about some of the pre-Covid activities we were able to do, the baby groups we visited, swimming and walks. We also said that we are sure that he will have questions when he is older and that our Letterbox contact would be a way of keeping in touch. We signed the letter 'From all of us' to maintain anonymity.

Later on this afternoon, we had a virtual call with our social workers. There are still significant delays with court proceedings. It was helpful to be able to speak about the settling in letter; as this is our first letter to his birth mother, we want to make sure we are doing it sensitively. We also wanted it to go on record that we still want to be able to meet her once Covid permits. We know that she wants to meet us, we just don't want it to get forgotten about as time goes on.

As we have gone through the process, our attitude to contact with the birth family shifted. I am sure we are not the only ones who are now sad that we haven't had the chance of meeting any birth family. Jessica and Mark also wanted the opportunity to meet their little one's birth parents – for this to be part of their story, and that of their little one.

> Contact was granted for the birth father every week, and the birth mother fortnightly. Our social worker suggested using a pay-as-you-go SIM card, which worked well. I switched on the phone at

the allotted times and switched it off in between. This provided an element of control for us. As the weeks went on with no contact I asked permission to send videos in our time window. It became clearer and clearer that the birth parents were unable to maintain regular contact, and my thoughts turned to the boy's life story. I felt a little cheated by the lack of contact. In training they'd talked of meeting up, chatting about family traits, the children's birth stories and even having a photo of everyone together. I went from hoping they wouldn't ring, to hoping they would. Either way we had no contact from either parent.

When the Placement Order was granted they didn't attend court. It was a virtual hearing on Skype, and in their absence it went straight to a final hearing. While part of me felt relieved that we weren't being challenged by the birth parents, part of me felt heartbroken for our boys. As time progresses and we navigate our way through the legal process, the stories we tell our children become more and more important.

We welcomed the chance to meet birth grandparents and siblings, and have added to our boys' memory boxes with care. We feel incredibly protective of their start in life, and responsible for making sure they grow up feeling comfortable with their story.

(Jessica and Mark, Early Permanence Placement/
Foster to Adopt, twin boys, 12 days old)

Every aspect of the adoption process has been impacted by Covid – from training to assessments, introductions, social worker visits and courts. Of course, our own process has been delayed and our opportunity to meet with Jake's birth mother was impacted, with our Local Authority not able to support face-to-face final contact sessions during the lockdown. Fortunately for Louise and Ian, their Local Authority was able to facilitate a Covid-secure final contact meeting:

Once the Placement Order was granted, Poppy's social worker arranged for contact to be reduced and finally stopped. The final 'Wish you well' contact sessions were arranged for late March. These sessions were impacted by lockdown and were postponed.

During lockdown, we had our Matching Panel and applied for our Adoption Order. The IRO at the LAC Review wanted to make sure that the 'Wish you well' contact sessions happened before the adoption hearing, so they took place in July. The sessions were risk assessed and we all had to agree to certain conditions such as wearing PPE. These final sessions will be important for Poppy in the future, although at the time she did not settle well.

(Louise and Ian, Foster to Adopt, girl, three months)

1 June

Jake's birthday card from his birth mother arrived today. As we had been pre-warned that we may find it upsetting, I had prepared myself for the worst. However, it was a lovely card and she had written him a message. We have put the card in a safe place and, hopefully, this will be the first of many, which along with the Letterbox correspondence we can share with him when he is old enough to understand.

9 June

Another social worker meeting today, again via video call. Once again, there were no particular updates and no progress with court dates. We spent most of the time talking about the Later Life letter which his social worker is going to give to him. This is a letter written from his social worker directly to him, explaining her role in the decisions that were made when he was a baby. This will be an honest account of the circumstances that led to his adoption. His social worker is hoping to work on the letter soon and will send me a draft when it is done. We have asked if it can be handwritten, rather than typed. There is something much more personal about a handwritten letter and I think this would be appropriate. She thought this was a lovely idea and has agreed.

We also spoke about his second life story book. I have to say I found this book harder to make. It was difficult to get the language right, appropriate for a six year-old to understand, building on the first book. It also made me feel emotional. I can see why life story work is so important and why we need to be open and honest from the beginning. We want to be there to support Jake as he grows up with his story.

Contact with birth siblings is another aspect of the Fostering for Adoption process which some families facilitate, again an important aspect of life story work. Charlotte and Richard reflect on their contact sessions with older siblings. At these sessions they experienced, first-hand, the impact that separating siblings can have on children:

> Little Brother had several court mandated contacts with his older siblings. We were present during these sessions, acting as facilitators. Given the age of the older siblings, one of us needed to care for Little Brother during these visits. We found these sessions hard, emotionally – we saw first-hand the love they had for each other and the devastation caused due to separation.
>
> (Charlotte and Richard, Foster to Adopt, siblings, weeks apart, one from foster care and a baby from hospital)

Adopters may be encouraged to develop relationships with siblings who have also been adopted. Louis and Nellie share their experience of phone calls, birthday cards and presents and their plans for meeting up at a time when the children are ready:

> A key consideration with our match would be that Jess would have contact with her older siblings – of course we didn't hesitate, they were her birth family. The siblings have been placed with their adoptive parents but they don't live near to us. Jess's social worker passed on our number and they got in touch and introduced themselves. We communicated via text, asking questions and sharing photos. The siblings sent Jess a gift to say 'Hello'; they were really excited to hear they had a baby sister – we have since shared birthday cards and presents. After getting to know them via text, we had a video call as parents. It was meant to be a quick 'Hi' but it lasted for two and a half hours – we got on so well. We agreed that we would go at the pace of the siblings as they were older and would need more preparation for a potential meeting. We continue to text, share photographs and video calls. We plan to meet as soon as we can (given the current Covid restrictions) – if it wasn't for lockdown we would have most definitely met already. From the very beginning the social workers emphasised the importance of this sibling

relationship. It has been positive so far and we can't wait to introduce the children to each other.

(Nellie and Louis, Early Permanence Placement, girl, three months)

There are some ongoing cases where direct contact with the birth parents is recommended to be of benefit for the child. Several of the families in this book have said that there are plans in place, post-Adoption Order, to be in direct contact with birth parents. Charlotte and Richard plan to have individual contacts once per year with the birth mum and older siblings, where they are hoping that this becomes a positive and safe arrangement going forward. Elaine and James also explain that in Northern Ireland, it is not unusual for face-to-face contact with birth parents to be set up as a post-adoption contract between all parties – of course, with the caveat that it is in the best interests of the child and safe to do so.

10 June

Every day, I go for a walk around the block with Jake. He has just started to walk, holding our hand. We stop every few metres, take a look at the leaves, the cracks in the walls and moss on the pavement. Our route takes us a whole hour, to walk what would usually take ten minutes. I am loving my Adoption Leave; life has really slowed down and I am appreciating these little, lovely moments with Jake.

This afternoon the health visitor rang. They are unable to do home visits at the moment, so instead, we received a phone call. We talked about dropping Jake's morning nap – at the moment he isn't really showing any of the key signs; he loves his sleep. She reassured me that this is fine and to follow Jake's lead – he will let us know when he is ready to drop it.

When we first met Jake, we were told by his foster carers that '*he is a happy, calm, content but serious baby.*' For the first few months, we would agree; it took quite a lot for him to smile freely. In the last month or so he is turning into a little comedian, mostly laughing at himself. His big smile, silly faces and giggles are never far away. Recently he has also become very loveable, wanting hugs from us both – he wraps his arms around our necks and snuggles in – just perfect.

29 June

Today was our reallocated court date. As predicted we have had no news, so more waiting. We are getting frustrated now and increasingly anxious; we are so worried about his birth parents contesting the adoption. We can't relax until the Adoption Order is granted. We really feel we were unprepared for this. We had no idea that birth parents are able to contest the adoption at this late stage in the process.

CHAPTER 10

OUR STORY CAN CONTINUE: TWO LEGALLY BECOMES THREE

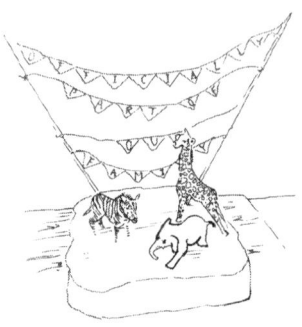

This is the final chapter, where Little J officially becomes part of our family. As you will read, we were kept in limbo right until the very end. However, we can now say we are parents to a beautiful (I know most parents say this about their children, but he really is so handsome), calm, funny and content little boy. After years of waiting and hoping our dreams have come true.

Since he has been with us he has taught us more than we could ever have imagined – about parenthood, play, life and, above all, about love.

2 July

Today my phone rang, a call from an unknown number. The person on the other end of the line began by saying *'Hello, this is Pam from Children's Social Services team. I understand that you have Jake in your care?'* My heart sunk and I felt sick. My first thought was *'they want him back.'* With sweaty palms, I confirmed that *'yes'* we do have Jake in our care.

She then proceeded to explain that she was from the medical team and she was ringing to book in another Looked After Child medical for him. I breathed a sigh of relief. *'Was that it?'* I thought.

I explained that his case was due in court soon for the final hearing, so perhaps it might not be needed. She said she would look into it and get back to me. Surely there are better ways to begin a phone call to an adoptive parent who is on tenterhooks waiting for news?

3 July

My granny, the centre of my family and my world, died today. For the past few months, due to Covid, we have only been able to see her through a window in her care home. It has been tough but she knew we were there, she even managed a smile for Little J.

One of the last things my grandpa said to me just before he died was *'Please look after Granny'* – and we did, right until the very end. If I take anything away from how sad I am feeling right now, it is how important grandparents are in the lives of children. My hope for Little J is that he has a special relationship with his grandparents, as I did mine.

11 July

Today we met up for a walk with our good friends. This is the first time we have seen them since going into lockdown in March. We had been waiting for a lovely moment to ask them to be Jake's Godparents, today was the day. They both cried, delighted to be asked. Like our other best friends, we know that they will be there for Jake, no matter what. He will grow up knowing that he is loved by them and can talk to them about anything.

27 July

We have got a big day tomorrow; Jake's case is in court. His social worker called and was optimistic that everything would be fine. We should hear tomorrow if the adoption is going to be contested by his birth family. If not, we will be given a date for the final court hearing where they will issue us with an Adoption Order, confirmation that we are his legal parents. With the delays due to Covid, this date really feels like a long time coming. Fingers crossed that after tomorrow there will be no more bumps in the road.

28 July

The case was in court at 10am this morning. As we waited we kept ourselves busy. We had a call from our social worker at 11:30am with news. There is yet more uncertainty. So far, the adoption has not been contested by his birth parents – but given that they haven't heard anything either way, they are not actually sure if they have received the legal paperwork. Given this, the judge has ordered that the court paperwork is hand-delivered to their last known address and to give the family another seven days to appeal. If there is no appeal within this seven-day period, then the final hearing will take place. At this time, we will hear the outcome of the appeals and the judge will decide if there is enough evidence to be able to grant the Adoption Order. We are now beginning to lose our nerve.

As adopters this is so upsetting. We have now had Jake in our care for nearly nine months and right up to this point we have had no agency in the process. We are very much the last people to hear any news. We are left hanging, right until the bitter end.

29 July

Jake and I had a playdate today with our good friends who we have met through adoption. It was so lovely to see them and for our boys to play together. We chatted about the practicalities, the emotion and of course the pure joy of adoption. We are so lucky that we have met this family; hopefully, our boys will grow up knowing each other, and be able to speak openly about adoption.

Despite starting the process together, going through the training and assessment at the same time, being approved at panel within a week of each other and both doing Fostering for Adoption, our experiences have been very different. Obviously unlike our experience, they adopted a sibling group from the beginning, while we were keen on a one-child placement. Like us, Elaine and James were matched with one child. However, in the case study below they share their experience of repeat adopting. On the same day they were approved to adopt their second child, as if by pure fate, they heard that their child's birth mother was due to have another baby:

> We were matched with our little one in May 2016, she came home in June 2016 and in January 2018 we formally adopted her. We decided

soon after that we were ready to go again and started our second assessment in May 2018. In April 2019 we were approved as adopters by the ADM. The same day we heard that our little one's birth mother was due to have another baby – that week. A week later our second baby came home to us.

(Elaine and James, Concurrent Placement from birth, a sibling to their three year-old)

1 August

We spent the day with my parents, having a lovely walk and picnic. It has been heart-wrenching not being able to spend time with them over recent months. I took a stunning photograph of my dad and Jake, standing at a fence – Jake looking up and my dad looking down – they adore each other. When my mum remarried after my birth father died, this extraordinary man took me under his wing. He taught and showed me that love is so much more than DNA. Now we have Little J in our lives, another relationship is blossoming. Jake is surrounded by love from both his nannies, his grandpa, grandad, honorary aunties and uncles – each playing a special part in his life.

6 August

We are on holiday at the moment. Given the Covid-19 restrictions, we have opted for a camping trip to Northumberland. As always, we had to get permission, informing the social workers which campsites we were staying at and making them aware of the Covid-safe restrictions in place with washing and eating facilities.

We are having such a wonderful time. Camping with Jake is both exhausting and amazing all wrapped up in one. This is what we dreamed of, having a little one to share our love of the outdoors with. He is teething at the moment which is making it a little unpredictable – touch wood, so far we haven't had too many dramas.

7 August

I spoke too soon with my entry yesterday. Last night was, hands-down, the worst night we have had so far with Jake. He woke up at 3am screaming; when I say screaming, I mean it. Nothing would console him. After 15 minutes, we decided to decamp to the car, by this point we must have woken up the entire campsite. Will sat in the car with him and tried to rock him to sleep. We decided we would do shifts, so I went back to the tent but just lay there. At 4:30am I went back out to check on them both. Will with a glazed expression was still rocking Jake; he on the other hand was wide awake and smiling. By 5am it was getting light. To give Will a break, I took Jake for a walk in the carrier down to the beach. We watched the sunrise, it was beautiful. By 8am I was back and we had given Jake his breakfast; the rest of the campers were emerging from their tents. It was soon time for Jake to go back to bed. He was ready for a nap and, given the events of the night, so were we. We definitely needed it; the three of us woke up at 11am, with the sun shining into the tent. We emerged to find all the tents immediately surrounding us gone – oh dear. I guess there is only one thing worse than a teething baby: a teething baby while camping.

10 August

I have been so sad today, it was granny's funeral. Will's parents came to the crematorium to look after Jake while we were in the service. Sadly, there were lots of restrictions in place, so the funeral was not what it should have been. There were limits on the number of people, so there was only immediate family, just eight of us. We all had to wear masks, sit two metres apart, no singing and no lingering or chatting afterwards. In the lead up to the funeral this had upset me. However, once we were in our seats, the eight of us, with the coffin, sitting overlooking the rolling fields in the sunshine, there was something lovely about the intimacy of it. Over the years, I have been to many funerals with granny and as I sat there I thought to myself that perhaps those shared experiences are more important than the event today. I also thought about her rolling her eyes and laughing about the fact she was having to have a slimmed-down Covid-19 funeral.

I am so grateful that she got to meet our Little J. I have heard it said that babies help people with dementia, and I have to say there was a twinkle in her eye each time she saw him.

The mobile granny bought me still hangs above Jake's cot. We have a ritual of blowing kisses to the figures and saying goodnight before bedtime – each time we do this, I think of my granny.

16 August

Today was a special day. We took Jake to buy his first pair of shoes. We had booked an appointment to have him measured and fitted. We came away with a gorgeous pair of navy leather shoes for toddlers taking their first steps and a card which said 'Baby's first shoes' – this will go in his memory box. We went to a lovely café for a celebratory lunch, just perfect.

Will soon goes back to work full time, having been working from home since the beginning of lockdown. When Jake arrived, Will had the standard two weeks of leave. We could never have dreamed that we would have had the opportunity for the three of us to spend six months together as a family unit. While Covid has been so terrible in many ways, we can't be anything other than grateful for this extra time we have had together.

17 August

Our health visitor came to see us today. This is the first time she has been to our house since lockdown began in March. Given Jake's 'Looked After Child' status, she said he was high up on the list for visiting. She came equipped with her visor, gloves and apron – despite the barriers, we had a lovely catch up. She is really pleased with his progress. He is keeping a good weight and is meeting his developmental milestones. At the end of the meeting, I gave her a card to say thank you for all she has done for us since Jake arrived. She cried and said *'nobody ever says thank you to health visitors'.* From Day 1 she offered us the reassurance we needed as new parents. She taught us to listen to our baby, rather than comparing to what others are saying or doing; she calmed me down when I was panicking; she was so supportive of the Fostering for Adoption process; she came to our LAC Reviews; and above all, she was caring.

Early on in the adoption process, our agency made it clear that the primary carer would need to take a year of Adoption Leave. At the time, Will and I talked about sharing the leave but generally, it was preferred that one parent becomes the main carer, for attachment building. We decided that I would take the full year. We can now see how it would be possible that you could have a whole year of Adoption Leave without the certainty of an Adoption Order. In a few days, we are hoping that Jake will be granted his Adoption Order and we will legally become his parents. Emotions have once again started to ramp up.

This book has charted the emotional burden of Fostering for Adoption, navigating the process and the uncertainty. In the case study below, Beatrix and Thomas speak about living with the fear of the unknown throughout the process and what it feels like once you have made it to the other end – the day your Adoption Order is granted.

> The not knowing was the hardest part of the process. You have to tell yourself they are not going to go back, and that this is forever. You get attached from the very first time you see their beautiful faces. If they had gone back it would have been absolutely devastating; as soon as they are with you, you start building a bond, your first picture, the day baby S met baby K and so on, so many memories. As soon as you get that phone call to say the court has made the final Adoption Order you just cry because you know that's it. Your dreams as a couple have come true and you have your forever family; it is so special, something to be treasured.
>
> (Beatrix and Thomas, Foster to Adopt, S five days old, K 22 months, siblings)

1 September

Tomorrow Jake's case is in court. Even though we are now so near to the end of the process, we are still kept hanging. For reasons I can't explain because they are too close to Little J's story, we don't yet know with much degree of certainty that the Adoption Order will be granted tomorrow. We are living on a knife-edge.

When we began the process, we certainly didn't realise that the decisions could still go either way this far down the line. We have now had Jake in our lives for nearly 11 months and we can't imagine life without him. As I shared with you early on in the book, when we began our journey we read the CoramBAAF (2017, p 5) document which states that Fostering for Adoption *'is not for the fainthearted or overly emotional'*. Having read our account, I don't think I need to tell you that I wear my heart on my sleeve and would certainly put myself in the 'emotional' category. The process is challenging – it is the not-knowing, right up to the very end. However, Will has been the calming influence and we have done this together.

We now have one more sleep until we find out the outcome; either this will be the end of the process and we will be celebrating or there will be more waiting. Either way, we know that all of this is being done in the best interests of Jake and for that we are grateful.

At 8pm tonight I had a feeling; just in case of a positive outcome tomorrow, I should make a cake. Three hours later and we now have a beautiful celebration cake. Fingers crossed all goes to plan tomorrow.

2 September

Written in the morning: Today is the day. In less than two hours we will know if today is the start of the rest of our lives together.

Written in the evening: We have been celebrating. This morning Little J officially became part of our family. There have been lots of happy tears and excitement in our house today. Finally, we can call him ours. From Day 1, he has been showered with love from all of our friends and family; we had so many calls to make to share the news. We couldn't have got through it without all of these people.

Our parents were on standby for an afternoon celebration. We were able to eat the 'just in case' celebration cake, topped with bunting which said 'Officially part of our family'. A perfect afternoon, the six of us raising a glass to Little J.

Despite the celebrations, however, there is a tinge of sadness. Our happiness is coming from a sad situation and this will stay with us forever. The day Jake came into our lives we made a promise to him. We will be open with him about his story and hold his hand as he navigates his journey through life – whatever happens, as his parents we will be there for him.

Tonight we ended the celebrations by reading him the story that we read to him on his first night with us. The story ends:

> *Our kisses are colours, and raindrops that flow, and pebbles, and acorns, and comets that glow, and flowers, and snowflakes that fall from above; they're our way, sweet baby to give you our love.*
>
> (Lawler, 2011)

It brings a tear to my eye every time.

3 September

This morning we woke up as Little J's forever mummy and daddy. The enormity of what we have been through over the past year has hit me. Before Jake woke up, Will and I lay in bed and hugged each other. We had done it; the little boy sleeping in his cot next door was ours.

To celebrate the three of us went on a special trip. On our panel day in May 2019, coincidently the day Little J was also born, we visited an independent book shop to calm our nerves before heading to the council office. Nearly sixteen months on, with our Adoption Order behind us, the three of us returned.

We asked the owner for a book recommendation and she directed us to *All Kinds of Families* (Hen, 2020). It is a beautiful book about the foundation of family, presented through different kinds of caring relationships that animals have with young babies – they all have one thing in common – *love*.

If I had known this time last year that it was possible to love a little one as much as this, I need not have worried. He is the centre of our world and we would move mountains for him.

Epilogue

I hope that you have finished this book knowing more about the Fostering for Adoption process and some of what it can entail for adopters. Throughout, you will have got a sense of the complexity of the process – one which involves social workers, judges, birth and adoptive parents, the foster carers, health care professionals and, of course, the child being at the centre of these relations. This account has been from our perspective as the adopters, to support others who are also considering this journey. While writing, I have tried to be empathetic to these processes, complexities and the emotions of Fostering for Adoption, for all involved.

Two weeks after our Adoption Order was granted, we decided to share our story. Our good news coincided with a leap of faith into the world of the adoption Instagram community; I set up an anonymous account and discovered a wonderful network of fellow adopters. I soon realised that this book could and should not be just about our story, so invited others to share their experiences of Fostering for Adoption. I was overwhelmed by the response and their willingness to share their stories of decision making, practicalities, emotions, contact and more. You will have got a sense from reading their stories that their backgrounds were diverse. While I haven't dwelled on difference in terms of sexuality, gender, race, ethnicity or disability, what the book shows is that diverse families had shared experiences which cut across difference – regardless of our backgrounds we all had shared emotions, sensitivities, hope and an openness to love.

It has been many months since the families sent me their case studies, so I felt it was appropriate to share where they now are on their journey. Receiving these updates, for me as an author, was emotional. I feel connected to these families and a real sense of privilege that they allowed me to share their story with you.

Hannah and Claire

Our eldest daughter was granted her Adoption Order at nine months old. She has been officially ours for nearly three years. She is progressing well and astounds us every day with how clever, smart and funny she is. Our youngest daughter moved in five months ago. There have been significant delays with court processes; so, we are eagerly awaiting her Adoption Order. Both girls had a very similar start in life and both are doing so well. As a family, we are now deciding whether we want a third addition, or a camper van – only time will tell.

Elaine and James

At the beginning of the summer holiday our Adoption Order was granted. We even managed to go to court and meet the judge, our children were so happy. Post-adoption with our first little one, we did Letterbox contact, but it was one sided. After the birth of the sibling, we were hopeful that we would be able to encourage the birth mother to engage and potentially move towards face-to-face contact; sadly due to circumstances, contact is no loner an option.

Charlotte and Richard

We recently had both Adoption Orders granted and can finally say that we are officially, legally a family. They are our sons, and we are their parents. Our boys are the most amazing little people we could ever have dreamt of. It is the greatest privilege to be called mama and daddy by them. What an incredible blessing to raise these gorgeous boys through the beauty of adoption. We never gave up. We think if you never give up you can make your dreams come true. They may change, look different than you imagined, different to almost everyone else you know but for us we wouldn't change anything now. We would do Fostering for Adoption again without hesitation. We often think if we had heard about experiences like ours prior to doing Fostering for Adoption, we would have been more concerned than we were. However, it has changed us for the better and we learnt that you don't know what you can take on until you are doing it. Fostering for Adoption is without a doubt worth the risk – adopting our boys has been the best thing we have ever done.

Sarah and Alex

We waited over a year to be matched and went through lots of heartbreak and false hope. After our failed relinquished baby, a few months later we were linked with a little girl. She was due to come home with us but at the eleventh hour we were informed that her auntie had come forward, and once again we were devastated. Despite these experiences, we have grown through our journey and surprised ourselves with how resilient we really are. Four months ago we accepted another Foster to Adopt placement; we are cherishing every smile, laugh and milestone. This has been the hardest thing we have ever done and we hope we are now on our way to our happy ending.

Nellie and Louis

We submitted our paperwork to the court in November 2020. Jess is doing amazingly well; she is meeting all of her milestones and is a very happy toddler. Our first Christmas together was a dream come true. In the New Year, we were anxious about not having news about a court date. Then we had a call to give us a day's warning for the court hearing. We received a phone call as soon as the judge had made the order. *'Congratulations mummy and daddy,'* our social worker said. We cried, we were so relieved. I scooped her up, gave her a kiss and told her she was staying with us forever. Of course, she was too young to understand, but one day she will. After all of our waiting, the six *'we have a baby to discuss'* conversations, and the failed links, we now know that all of that was meant to be. We are so happy.

Beatrix and Thomas

The Fostering for Adoption journey for us was hard but it was a risk we wanted to take. We believed that this was our time to become parents. All court proceedings are now complete and legally they are now our children. Holding their Adoption Orders in our hands was the best feeling in the world; these two beautiful children are now part of our forever family.

Katie and Jack

We were foster carers for our little one for four months. When his case went to court we were more nervous than when we went to Adoption Panel. Fortunately, his Placement Order was approved and the plan for our little one was adoption. Five days later we were officially matched. Since then we have submitted our application to adopt him and hopefully, it will only be a few more weeks until he will be officially ours. This has been a whirlwind of 12 months. We feel truly blessed that we are on our way to becoming his parents.

Rachel

Jack's Adoption Order was granted shortly before his second birthday. There were numerous delays with multiple court hearings. Both birth parents contested the Adoption Order application. Although this meant there were delays, I am pleased that Jack will know that he was loved and they wanted to care for him. He is doing so well, is settled and is a lovely little boy with heaps of energy. He is gentle, brave, kind and funny (and a hundred other wonderful things), rounded off with having the most beautiful smile.

I am so pleased that I decided to do Fostering for Adoption, even with the challenges it has involved. If Jack and I had been matched via the traditional pathway to adoption, I am sure he would have been 11 months at the earliest. He would have experienced both the loss of his birth family and the loss of a foster family. I feel so lucky that I met him as a tiny baby and I was able to protect him from another move. I am privileged to be his mummy and I can't wait for our next adventures together. I love him more than I could possibly ever explain.

Joanne and John

Our Adoption Order was granted in February 2020, weeks before the country went into lockdown. We were so thankful that our court date fell when it did, so we didn't experience any delays due to Covid; however, it did mean we weren't able to celebrate with our family and friends or have a Celebratory Hearing. We can't imagine life without our son and are so happy that we decided to grow our family through adoption.

Sam and Alexander

After nine months of waiting and uncertainty, we finally have our Placement Order for our little girl. All relative reassessments came back negative. The little baby that came to us is now a little girl who is very much attached to us, as we are to her. Let's hope this Fostering for Adoption story ends in adoption.

Jessica and Mark

At the end of January, we had the amazing news from our social worker that our Adoption Order had been granted. The boys are now legally ours and officially share our family name. From the initial fast-paced movement of linking and placement, with added meetings for our little 'Looked After Children' – we felt the process slowed dramatically near the end. We now feel like a weight has been lifted, knowing that we have finally reached the last hurdle. Seeing our boys' social worker for the final time was emotional. She handed over their life story books and spent three hours telling us every piece of knowledge she had about their birth family. We will treasure this information, keeping it private and safe, until our little ones are ready to learn how they came to join our family.

Paul and John

For us, the whole experience was devastating; it really shook us to the core. Our dream had come true and then all hope was dashed within weeks. We had to continue to love and care for this baby that was highly likely to no longer be ours; these scars will remain with us forever.

We took some time out from everyone and everything to grieve and reset. We had counselling to deal with the loss. When the time was right, we re-started the process but as straightforward adopters. With our experience, this made us much more anxious going through the process, including right up until the final court hearing where our son officially became ours. I still advocate Early Permanence but would want others considering it to make sure they have the resilience to manage should the worst happen.

Nicole and Paulo

We were approved in December 2020. In the weeks before the panel, we were led to believe that matching could happen very soon, within weeks. This raised our expectations. Our Local Authority wanted us to wait three months before giving us access to Link Maker; there are currently no matches to our criteria locally. I am finding this wait incredibly difficult; it has triggered memories of trying to conceive – lots of waiting. I am trying not to be impatient but my journey to motherhood has taken close to 20 years, so with that in mind, maybe I am not so impatient. Whether we accept a child on Fostering for Adoption or through traditional adoption, we need to keep hoping it will happen soon.

Louise and Nick

Our Adoption Order has now been granted. Of course, there were some bumps in the road which we fully expected, but right now, none of that matters; our daughter is legally ours. We are over the moon and everything we went through has been worth it. She became our daughter the day we met her, but now she is legally ours. We recently received her certificate and we were hit by a wave of emotion as we read her name, followed by our surname. We would do it again in a heartbeat.

Louise and Ian

We are happy to say that our little one is now officially our child. The Adoption Order was granted just before her first birthday in September. She has now lived with us for 16 months and we are loving watching her grow and develop into a cheeky, happy little girl. We realise that we are very privileged to have seen many of her 'firsts'. We can't wait to be able to take her for her first swimming lesson, first haircut and first holiday.

Kristie

I have applied to the court for the Adoption Order and am currently waiting for a court date. The application was quite stressful as it was returned twice for more information, despite my social worker saying it was fine. I am keeping my fingers crossed that it will be straightforward with the final court decisions. Throughout the process, I was blessed that the risk was minimal. Birth mother withdrew from the social workers and said she wasn't able to care for the babies. For reasons I can't go into, the social worker team agreed to a name change. My biggest worry is that one day I may have to tell my babies that their birth mother has passed away due to her circumstances; if this happens we will work through it as a family. I would do Fostering for Adoption again in a heartbeat. The experience and time I had to bond with them from the early days outweighed the potential risk. The love that I have for my babies is more than I could have ever imagined and I would do anything for them; they are my world.

Taken as a collective, these stories show the resilience and hope that Fostering for Adoption carers have as they navigate the process. These stories have all been hard, really hard, and not all of them have ended how the adopters hoped. All these families took a risk, but ultimately they took the risk on behalf of the baby in their care. I am hugely indebted to each and every one of them for sharing their stories with me, and ultimately with you.

Now for the end of our story.

Looking back

Before we began the adoption process our lives were full, bursting at the seams. We had busy and demanding jobs, and volunteer responsibilities. We went on holidays, camped, climbed mountains, renovated our home and were zigzagging across the country catching up with friends and family. During our assessment, we were asked how we would fit in a child? How would they fit into our life and routine? The reason our life was so busy was because we had a child-shaped hole to fill. We took every opportunity going; this is how we coped.

We now have a two-year-old toddler and he is our priority. As we began the adoption process, nobody could have predicted that we would have been navigating this through a global pandemic. Entering lockdown with a young baby was tough (as I am sure many new parents will testify). At the time when I needed my mum the most, like many, we had to stick to the rules. Over a year since the first lockdown, we have only just stayed the night with my parents. We have missed out on so much – the family dinners, playing, bath time, cuddles, night-time kisses, early morning snuggles and more. We have a lifetime to catch up and we can't wait. While lockdown and Covid restrictions have been hard in so many ways, it has also been a blessing. Our life has slowed right down; six months of my parental leave was spent with Little J and Will at home – what a wonderful chance to bond as a family. We will treasure this time that we spent together. We want to remember those days that it took us an hour to walk around the block when Jake was taking his first steps, or the time spent at the allotment during lockdown and the long walks with him in the backpack. This is when life was on go slow, and I hope we take some of this with us as we move forward.

During our adoption assessment, a slight critique was voiced about our expectations of an adopted child. Our careers and ambition were seen as a potential negative, not by our assessing social worker, but by the system – we were warned that we may be questioned about this at the panel – pre-judged that we may have unrealistic expectations of a future little one. On several occasions, we challenged this. Yes, both of us are professionals, but from the beginning, we have been open to exploring all pathways for a child in our care and now that he is in our life we are now even more committed to supporting him in finding his future.

I often think back to the 'perfect child' exercise that we went through during our assessment. At the time, I was confused about why we were being asked to reframe our expectations of a child that may join our family. Now he is with us, we have changed our thinking. At the beginning of the process, the social workers have a duty of care to future children who may be placed – if adopters have unrealistic expectations of a future child this can lead to disappointment, disconnection and unfortunately in some cases, breakdown of placement. If this happens then ultimately the child will experience further emotional trauma. Going through the process opened our eyes to the impacts of abuse and trauma, but what matters the most is that for us, our Little J is perfect; he isn't a 'perfect child', because this doesn't exist. None of us are perfect; he is perfect because he is ours. As he grows up, like any parent, we will want what is best for him and guide him in the ways we feel are appropriate.

Fostering for Adoption has given us so much to be grateful for. It was because of this pathway to adoption that Little J was able to be placed with us so quickly after the court decision; within 24 hours we had begun introductions. We would have waited months if going through the standard adoption process. With a Placement Order in hand, our pathway was certainly less risky than other stories you have read in this book – however, it was still a Fostering for Adoption placement and we were well aware of the 'air of uncertainty'. Given the turbulent time we had in the matching phase, we didn't trust that it would all go through. We were nervous. Our social workers were professional and never promised anything, right up until the day of our Adoption Order.

It was on our introduction evening that we first heard about Fostering for Adoption. We had no idea that being placed with a baby could be an option. Everything we knew about adoption was about toddler placements and older. I will never forget the glance I gave to Will in that session. I was excited; this could be it, our chance of having a baby. He smiled back at me; we both felt this route could be for us. Our feelings about Fostering for Adoption were then cemented on Day 3 of our training. One of the other participants, reflecting on her own adoption, said that what upsets her the most, now as an adult, is that she has nobody in her life that knows her full story. Multiple moves as a baby and young child before being adopted meant that her story was fragmented and for her this hurt. From this moment I knew that I wanted to do Fostering for Adoption. I wanted us to be there from the beginning, to know the full story. Personally, this route to adoption also gave me hope that I would be able to have a newborn baby; I wanted the sleepless nights, the snuggles and everything in between. In fact, on reflection, prior to placement I pinned too much hope on being placed with a newborn. Much of the training and narrative around Fostering for Adoption was about newborn babies. When we heard about Jake, he was four months old. Deep down I knew this baby was for us, meaning from this point on we were not going to be able to care for a newborn.

As you have read, our journey to being placed with Jake was not easy. The anticipation, the let-down, the waiting, the decisions and emotional toil were really hard. However, I now realise that we had to go through all of those to get to our Little J. In the process of being chosen for other Fostering for Adoption newborn babies, we learnt a lot about the risk and the scenarios that potential adopters can be faced with. By the time we were told about our Little J, we had re-evaluated our priorities; we had been told that he was happy, healthy and content. Compared to the newborns that we had been offered which were withdrawing from various cocktails of drugs and with uncertainties around family permanence, this four-month-old, who could be placed on Fostering for Adoption, for us was a less risky option. What we have learnt from going through the process and from collating the stories in this book is that there are so many variables and circumstances – some riskier than others. I would encourage anyone who is considering this route to growing their family to be open-minded. Throughout the whole process, we thought we wanted a girl – after being told about and offered only boys, we were beginning to think that we were destined to have a boy in our family. I wish now that I had been more open-minded about this from the beginning – he is our world, our little boy.

One of the reasons I was so sad about not being placed with a newborn was that I wouldn't be there for the 'firsts' and I am sure many readers will resonate with this. I was sad that we would miss the first days, the middle of the night feeds, the first smile, the first roll; the list goes on. I wanted to be there for all of it. Am I over it? No, not really. I am still sad about not being there for him from the very beginning, the early days. In fact, now that I am his mummy, it makes me more upset as I wanted to be there for his full story. Jake came to us when he was still very much a baby; he needed us for everything. There were still firsts and we had the privilege of being there for so many of these – the first time he sat up, first tastes, first Christmas, first tooth, first crawl, first haircut, first painting, first steps, first words and so, so much more. However, I now know that whatever age you are placed with a child, six hours, six days, six weeks, six months or age six – there will be firsts. These firsts will be for you and your family – whether it be the first steps or the first time at school – these will be special times and you will treasure them.

There is a point in adoption which I am sure many families hold on to, the point where your child has been with you for longer than with anyone else. This moment is empowering because you realise that you know this child better than anyone. You know how he likes to sleep, what he likes to eat, what makes him cross or frustrated and how he likes to be comforted – it is an amazing feeling.

When I look back at the whole of our Fostering for Adoption experience, it was both wonderful and excruciating. Yes, it was emotional, scary and anxiety-inducing, but it was also the best decision we have ever made. Hand on heart we could not have got through it without our family, friends and each other. Throughout the process, we spoke openly about the challenges with my closest friends and our parents. we also made friends going through the process and we are thankful to those we met on our training course. I have spoken about one family in particular – the one who I made a beeline to on the first day of training. This was the start of our friendship. What I didn't realise at the time was that these friendships don't end when you have finished the training, go to panel, been through the matching process, the early days of placement or are waiting for Adoption Orders. These friendships are for the long haul; these are the people who truly 'get it' and always will.

During our training, like all adopters, we had to show we had done our research and reading about trauma, abuse, PACE and attachment; the social workers have to know that you understand that growing your family through adoption is not just a route to becoming parents. Often it is described as 'parenting plus'. We did our reading, dived into the recommended books written by adopters, read scientific journal articles about babies withdrawing from drugs and listened to podcasts by social workers, adopters, birth parents and adoptees. We felt prepared, ready for our assessment. However, I have the same feeling as I do when I read city guidebooks before going on a city break; I do the research but none of it really sinks in until we are there, in the moment, navigating the city, being there on the ground and getting stuck in. It is the same with adoption. I am now finding myself re-reading the books we read a few years ago and widening our resources; I want to know more – how I can support our son as he grows with us, his new family. I often think back to our training on PACE and find myself wanting to know more about trauma and attachment building (as a side note, yes, it is still a family joke that Will has trouble remembering the associated words). As Jake works his way through his toddler years, he will no doubt struggle with his emotions as he learns about his environment, lack of control and negotiation; we will take what we have learnt about therapeutic parenting and put these tools to work. During our training, we were told that the 'naughty step' approach to behaviour management should not be used uncritically – particularly for those children who have experienced trauma, abuse, abandonment and multiple placements. For these children, they may need 'time in' with their parent or caregiver to be calm, together – rather than be left to deal with their emotions on their own. We have made a 'mental note' of this for when the time comes.

There are other books that are on my reading list, those that are written by adopters and adoptees; some come as recommendations, others with trigger warnings saying that they are difficult but important to read. In time, when we are ready, we will read these books. We want to be informed and continue to learn how it is best to support our son as he grows up. When we started the adoption process, we were naive to think that adopting a newborn or young baby would reduce the risk of harm. However, through the training, assessment, the matching and placement we have become much more aware and educated about trauma, abuse and the potential impact on very young children. I often think back to the example we were told about in our training, of the baby who reacted to the smell in a fast-food restaurant being reminded of in utero trauma. Recently we had an experience with Jake that made us think about this. We were at Will's mum's house, a space where he is comfortable and feels safe. A plumber was fitting a new bathroom and Jake's reaction shocked us. Of course, with lockdown, he is not used to other people being in his safe spaces, only us as his parents and his grandparents for childcare – so yes, a stranger in the house would be frightening. However, he cried uncontrollably and wrapped his arms tightly around my neck, a tight grip, not wanting to let go. He took over an hour to comfort and calm down. On the one hand, his reaction was positive; he turned to us to keep him safe, our attachment is strong. However, his reaction also seemed disproportionate. Of course, we will never know if this was a trigger for him, but what we can do is be there for him, hug him tightly and tell him that we will keep him safe, always.

There has been another experience that is important to share. It only happened last week, during the final stages of completing the proofs for the book – it was so profound that we felt it needed to be shared. A package arrived from our foster carer and inside there were some special things. One of them was Rhino, a small, cuddly toy that was bought for Jake on their first visit to the zoo, aged seven weeks. When Jake came to us, Rhino stayed behind to take care of the foster carers' daughter who was very sad to see him leave their home. Recently the little girl decided that it was now time for Rhino to be returned. For context, Jake had this soft toy for three months. Over 18 months later, last week, they were reunited. It was quite something. Jake took one look at Rhino and from a look in his eyes and his reaction, we knew that he recognised Rhino. He took the toy from me, clutched it under his arm and said 'baby' – since, Rhino has been kept close, day and night. There is no doubt that Little J remembers Rhino; it has been incredible to watch the thread of attachment rebuild between these two. Rhino is here to stay; he is more than welcome in our family, and he is clearly very special. These two moments, with the plumber and Rhino, have really made us think about the prior experiences of very young babies – the power of moments, memories and emotions that stimulate both positive and negative responses.

Our perceptions and those of others

Since the day we sat down in the café in Norfolk and completed the online Expression of Interest form, we have changed as a couple, changed our perceptions of adoption but also more specifically of trauma, abuse, contact with birth family and more. In the beginning, contact scared us – of course, it still scares us, but that is more related to the unknown; what has changed is our openness to sharing our little one with others. Yes, Little J is now legally ours, in that we have vowed to keep him safe and guide him through life as part of our family. However, running through Jake's body is a connection that is beyond us as a couple, beyond Alice and Will.

Throughout this process, we have heard from social workers, adoptees, adopters (via books, social media, magazines, podcasts and personal communication) and one resounding message is that as adopters we need to be open to Jake, one day, asking us questions, wanting to know more and searching for his birth family. Now that we have Jake in our lives, I can't imagine this being any other way; we want to be there for him, we want to be the ones he asks those questions to, we want to make sure we normalise adoption in our family, so that he grows up knowing that we are there for him, whatever decisions he makes.

Once our Adoption Order was granted, we received Jake's Later Life letter. His social worker has written him the most beautiful, considered letter, explaining from her perspective why he was adopted. I cried. In it, she explained that he may not want to read it all at once and he may want someone to be with him when he chooses to read it. I hope with all my heart that he wants us to sit with him while he reads it. I want to say 'hold our hand' but I imagine he is going to be in his early adulthood and won't want to be holding hands with mummy and daddy. However, I also know that by the time he is ready, he will have other people in his life he can trust. Whoever he sits with, I just want him to know that we will be there for him. It is his story and we will treasure it.

I recently had my first Mother's Day, legally as a mother. Going through the process, I have to say I was naive in thinking that once we were matched and had a little one with us, that all future Mother's Days would be rosy, just perfect with our baby. Last year, once he had been placed I realised that this is far from reality. It is days like Mother's Day that are a raw reminder of everything we have been through to get to this stage of a little human calling me 'mamma'. We share our baby with another mummy – in words, feelings, actions and thoughts. I also think about his foster family. The pure love that they had for Little J will stay with me forever. At the end of transition week, my heart ached for the loss that the family were experiencing; I was unprepared for this and these feelings hit me hard. On the night before we brought Jake home, as I lay in bed sobbing, we made a promise to ourselves, that this family would be in our lives as he grows up. We didn't collect him from the hospital as a newborn, we don't know his full story, but we know the people that can piece together the early days. They are his beginning, the start of his story, and now they are part of our life too.

From time to time, the perceptions and comments of others still take me off guard. One that sticks with me was a comment about not being his real mummy. It was like a punch in the tummy; I felt sick. As Little J and I drove home, we sang 'Old McDonald had a farm' – I looked at his little face in the mirror and shed a tear. I am very much real; I am a real mummy. I looked up the definition of 'real'. The Oxford English Dictionary defines it as *'actually existing as a thing, not imagined or supposed ... genuine'.* I am his real and genuine mummy. He is special because he has two mummies, two very real mummies. He will always be my baby and I will always be his very real mummy. I also think that as new adopters, we put pressure on ourselves and are constantly thinking that we are being watched and judged. In the early days of being placed with a child, you and they are in survival mode – take one day at a time and learn how to be with one another and try not to think about being under the watchful eye of friends, family, social services and, of course, wider society.

Despite the few comments or the awkward conversations, our family and wide network of friends and colleagues have been with us from the beginning. The support we have received has blown us away and we will forever be grateful for this. At Christmas this year, our first as an official family, one of our friends sent us a card, addressed to 'Alice, Will and Jake'. She then drew an arrow to the comma and wrote:

> It makes me so happy to write this comma. Who knew punctuation could do so much.

A comma is so simple, it is a single mark on a page, a small line between two words. It is small, but powerful – and for us, unites our family of three.

It is these small acts of kindness which mean so much; our friendships have deepened and grown throughout this process and we thank each and every one of them. If you are reading this book because you have a family member, or perhaps a good friend, starting the Fostering for Adoption process, then I hope that you have picked up a few tips on how you can support them. It will be hard, but if you show them you care, can listen and be open to new ways of thinking about family and love, then I am sure you will be doing just fine.

Love

Prior to starting the adoption process, one of my main anxieties was about love. This escalated as we made our way through the process and was particularly at the forefront of my mind during the matching and waiting phase. *What if this little one didn't love us? What if we didn't bond?* I remember having conversations with Will about love. I would lie in bed at night and come out with questions like *'I didn't know you and now I love you, so surely adoption is similar?'* There is the potential to love someone unconditionally, without blood ties. As I sit here writing the end of this book, what I now know is that I needn't have worried. Within a week of Jake living with us, as you would have read, he went off for his final contact session with his birth mother. He was collected by a social worker. This was the moment I knew that I was in love with him. I knew that I would love him unconditionally whatever the outcome. I knew that I wanted his final contact session to go as well as it could; I knew that I would do anything for him, always. This was week one and I just knew that I loved him.

Last week, our Little J ended up being taken to the hospital – a scary moment for any parent. As I sat with him in the ambulance, blue lights flashing, I held his hand. I went into a trance-like state, watching him breathe; as his mummy I knew his body best. When we were at the hospital, I was able to answer the doctors' questions related to how long he had been unwell for, what he had eaten, when we had last given him medicine – but there was one question I couldn't answer – about his birth. I didn't know the answer and probably never will. Did this bring a wave of sadness over me? Yes, of course, but then something beautiful happened. The nurse who was standing by us looked into my eyes and I knew then that she got it. She understood. In a quiet moment later, she explained that her daughter was now 25 – she adopted her as a young baby. A smile between us was exchanged, nothing more needed to be said. As

I cradled our little one through the night on the ward I thought about love and can say this – for anyone at the start of your journey, or awaiting placement – love happens and it grows within and between every moment of every day.

Through our little one we are connected to two people who we have never met. It makes me sad that we didn't get the chance to meet them. Much of the content in this book presents birth parents in the context of contact sessions where the focus is on the procedures and logistics and the adopters' emotional experiences. Given that this book is about the process, this possibly isn't surprising. It is my hope that in the months and years to come stronger threads of connection will emerge between our little one and his birth parents – they are his, in a way that my husband and I never will be. When we think about love we cannot do anything other than saying that we have an openness to love his birth family as they are the ones that produced this wonderful human being that we now call our son. As the years go on and we hopefully exchange letters, we will come to know more, have an opportunity to ask questions and importantly share our love for Little J.

On the eve of starting our Fostering for Adoption placement, there were so many 'what ifs' – *what if the plans change tomorrow and it is called off? What if the foster carers don't like us? What if we don't know what to do with a baby? What if we don't bond?* This list was endless. Now we are out the other side, I know that the stars were aligned and we were meant to be together, forever. You have to believe that you are in this together, you have to hold on tight and ride the waves of uncertainty and hope that your lives together can continue. We began this journey on 4 September 2018, when we sat in the council office attending the information evening; eight months and three days later we went to Adoption Panel in the hope that we would be approved as adoptive parents. In another five months and 26 days, we woke up knowing that would be the day we would meet our Little J. He then lived with us, first on a Fostering for Adoption placement and then on an Adoptive Placement for ten months and two days until his Adoption Order was granted. This journey took 23 months and 30 days – over these years, months and days we have learnt so much about ourselves – about acceptance, belonging, identity and most of all about love. People often exclaim at the amount of time it takes to become parents through adoption – yes, we agree, there were periods where we felt like our time would never come and there were the inevitable delays due to the pandemic – but overwhelmingly we have the sense that, for us, this time was important – for us to learn how to be parents via adoption and for us to be matched with our Little J.

I can't talk about love without mentioning our immediate family – our parents. They have been with us every step of the way throughout this process. For them, they were not only supporting us as their daughter and son – but they too were taking a leap into the unknown. They were agreeing to support and love this child, unconditionally. They read the books, went on the training, spoke to others in their position – they were ready. What they probably were not ready for was the overwhelming feeling of love they have for this small child. It is a pleasure to watch their bond develop and both Will and I are forever grateful for the support and love they have shown to us and Jake.

This has been the hardest, most emotional, anxiety-inducing time of our life, but it was also the best decision we have ever made. With Fostering for Adoption we took the risk, and for us it was a risk worth taking. On New Year's Day 2020, when we sat reviewing his paperwork for the Matching Panel, our eyes fixed on to his date and time of birth – Little J was born on the same day, at the same time that we were in our panel meeting to become parents – for us, this was meant to be. No, we weren't there from the very beginning as we so hoped we would be, but as he grows from a toddler, young child, young person, to adult, together we will tell our story of how we came to be a family. Yes, Fostering for Adoption is risky, yes, it is uncertain, but it can also be the start of something beautiful.

This book has been about our journey through the Fostering for Adoption process and has been carefully crafted to not disclose the details of Little J's story – for this is his story, not ours, to share. We end this book where we began, with the blue box in his room. This box holds his belongings, his treasures and his story – his past, present and future.

For us, as Alice, Will and Jake – our story as a family of three has just begun.

References

Adoption UK (2015) The Wall. [online] Available at: www.slideshare.net/AdoptionUK/the-wall-53186287 (accessed 23 April 2021).

AFA Cymru (2016) Foster to Adopt: Practice Guidance. [online] Available at: www.afacymru.org.uk/wp-content/uploads/2019/10/NASF2Afinal.pdf (accessed 24 June 2021).

Broadhurst, K, Alrouh, B, Mason, C, Ward, H, Holmes, L, Ryan, M and Bowyer, S (2018) *Born into Care: Newborn Babies Subject to Care Proceedings in England*. Nuffield Foundation, London: The Nuffield Family Justice Observatory.

Brown, R and Mason, C (2021) *Understanding Early Permanence: A Small-scale Research Study*, Final Report from the Centre for Child and Family Justice Research. Lancaster University. [online] Available at: www.cfj-lancaster.org.uk/app/nuffield/files-module/local/documents/Early%20Permanence%20Brown%20and%20Mason%20FINAL%20March%202021%20LAUNCH.pdf (accessed 25 April 2021).

Children Act (1989) Legislation. Section 1: Welfare of the Child. [online] Available at: www.legislation.gov.uk/ukpga/1989/41/part/I (accessed 3 June 2021).

Children and Families Act (2014) Legislation: c 6. [online] Available at: www.legislation.gov.uk/ukpga/2014/6/notes/division/2 (accessed 30 March 2021).

Coram (2021a) About Us. [online] Available at: www.coram.org.uk/about-us (accessed 31 March 2021).

Coram (2021b) Adopting a Baby: Early Permanence. [online] Available at: www.coramadoption.org.uk/adoption-process/children-waiting-adoption/adopting-baby-early-permanence (accessed 1 April 2021).

Coram and BAAF (2013) Fostering for Adoption: Becoming a Carer. [online] Available at: www.coram.org.uk/sites/default/files/resource_files/47%20Fostering%20for%20Adoption%20leaflet%20%28carers%29_2013.pdf (accessed 24 June 2021).

CoramBAAF (2017) *Fostering for Adoption: A Child-centred Solution – Guide for Prospective FfA Carers*. [online] Available at: www.first4adoption.org.uk/wp-content/uploads/2013/06/Fostering-for-Adoption-Carers-leaflet-2017.pdf (accessed 30 March 2021).

CoramBAAF (2018) *Child's Permanence Report (CPR)/Annex B Report, Guidance Notes and Additional Resources*. [online] Available at: https://corambaaf.org.uk/sites/default/files/electronic-forms/SAMPLE%20CoramBAAF%20Form%20CPR%202018.pdf (accessed 30 March 2021).

CoramBAAF (2021) *Statistics: England, Looked after Children, Adoption and Fostering Statistics for England*. [online] Available at: https://corambaaf.org.uk/fostering-adoption/looked-after-children-statistics/statistics-england#:~:text=During%20year%20ending%2031%20March,partnership%2C%20married%20or%20neither (accessed 30 March 2021).

Department for Education (2011) *An Action Plan for Adoption: Tackling Delay*. [online] Available at: https://assets.publishing.service.gov.uk/government/uploads/system/uploads/attachment_data/file/180250/action_plan_for_adoption.pdf (accessed 30 March 2021).

Department for Education (2013) *Further Action on Adoption: Finding More Loving Homes*. [online] Available at: https://assets.publishing.service.gov.uk/government/uploads/system/uploads/attachment_data/file/219661/Further_20Action_20on_20Adoption.pdf (accessed 30 March 2021).

Dibben, E and Howorth, V (2017) *The Role of Fostering for Adoption in Achieving Early Permanence for Children*. CoramBAAF. [online] Available at: https://earlypermanence.org.uk/wp-content/uploads/The-role-of-Fostering-for-Adoption-in-achieving-early-permanence-for-children.pdf (accessed 30 March 2021).

Donovan, S (2013) *No Matter What: An Adoptive Family's Story of Hope, Love and Healing*. London: Jessica Kingsley Publishers.

Families for Children (2021) *Fostering to Adopt*. [online] Available at: https://familiesforchildren.org.uk/fostering-to-adopt/ (accessed 29 March 2021).

First4Adoption (2021) *Adoption Glossary*. [online] Available at: www.first4adoption.org.uk/being-an-adoptive-parent/adoption-glossary/ (accessed 30 March 2021).

Hen, S (2020) *All Kinds of Families*. London: Red Shed.

Hughes, D (2021) The Attitude: Playfulness – Acceptance – Curiosity – Empathy. [online] Available at: www.danielhughes.org/p.a.c.e..html (accessed 23 April 2021).

Human Rights Act (1998) Legislation: Article 8, Right to Respect for Private and Family Life. [online] Available at: www.legislation.gov.uk/ukpga/1998/42/schedule/1/part/I/chapter/7 (accessed 3 June 2021).

Lawler, J (2011) *If Kisses Were Colours*. London: Templar.

Laws, S, Wilson, R and Rabindrakumar, S (2012) Concurrent Planning Study: Interim Report. [online] Available at: www.coram.org.uk/sites/default/files/resource_files/Concurrent%20Planning%20Study%202012.pdf (accessed 30 March 2021).

NHS (2021) Foetal Alcohol Syndrome. [online] Available at: www.nhs.uk/conditions/foetal-alcohol-syndrome/ (accessed 23 April 2021).

RCPCH (2018) Health and Social Care Committee: Inquiry into the First 1000 days of Life. Response submitted by the Royal College of Paediatrics and Child Health. [online] Available at: www.rcpch.ac.uk/sites/default/files/2018-09/first_1000_days_-_rcpch_response_-_final.pdf (accessed 31 March 2021).

Sandman, C A and Davis, E P (2012) Neurobehavioural Risk is Associated with Gestational Exposure to Stress Hormones. *Expert Review of Endocrinology & Metabolism*, 7(4): 445–59.

Shukla, S, Zirkin, L B and Pomar, E G (2020) Perinatal Drug Abuse and Neonatal Drug Withdrawal. [online] Available at: www.ncbi.nlm.nih.gov/books/NBK519061/ (accessed 12 August 2021).

The Adoption (Northern Ireland) Order (1987) Freeing for Adoption. [online] Available at: www.legislation.gov.uk/nisi/1987/2203/part/III/crossheading/freeing-for-adoption (accessed 3 June 2021).

UK Government (2021) Reporting Year 2020: Children Looked After in England Including Adoptions. [online] Available at: https://explore-education-statistics.service.gov.uk/find-statistics/children-looked-after-in-england-including-adoptions (accessed 30 March 2021).

West Berkshire Council (2021) Fostering for Adoption, Temporary Approval as Foster Carers of Approved Prospective Adopters, West Berkshire Children's Services Procedures Manual. [online] Available at: www.proceduresonline.com/westberks/cs/p_foster_for_adopt.html (accessed 30 March 2021).

Zero to Three (2017) Still Face Experiment Dr Edward Tronick. [online] Available at: www.youtube.com/watch?v=YTTSXc6sARg (accessed 7 November 2020).

Index

Adoption Leave, xiii, 2, 5, 11, 20, 28, 49, 51, 71, 90, 94, 95, 118, 121, 188, 195
adoption notebook, 20
Adoption Order (AO), xiii, xviii, 2, 3, 12, 14, 15, 20, 21, 114, 146, 153, 160, 172, 177, 178, 179, 180, 181, 182, 183, 184, 185, 186, 187, 188, 191, 192, 195, 196, 198, 199, 200, 201, 202, 203, 204, 206, 209, 214
Adoption Panel, xiii, 25, 38, 42, 43, 44, 45, 46, 47, 48, 49, 50, 51, 52, 53, 54, 55, 56, 57, 58, 59, 60, 61, 62, 63, 64, 65, 66, 67, 68, 69, 70, 71, 72, 94, 95, 96, 159, 163, 201, 214
Adoption Placement, 8, 9, 11
Adoption Placement Report (APR), 160
Agency Decision Maker (ADM), xiii, 36, 69, 87, 113, 146, 161, 193
An Action Plan for Adoption: Tackling Delay, 5
attachment, 8, 20, 31–3, 38, 44, 51, 53, 56, 67, 90, 110, 169, 173, 175, 180, 183, 209–10

birth parents, 2, 3–4, 6–9, 10–12, 28, 34, 38–9, 44, 46–9, 56, 80, 101, 110, 111, 113–15, 129, 141–5, 184–6, 188, 211, 214

Care Order (CO), xiii, 44, 119
Celebratory Hearing, xiii, 88, 93, 94, 114, 115

Child Permanence Report (CPR), xiv, 32, 35, 39, 54, 154, 157, 158, 164, 166
Children's Services, 109
Concurrent Care Placement, 141
Concurrent Planning, xiv, 3, 4, 5, 6, 7
court proceedings, 2, 4, 44, 113, 160, 161, 178, 184

direct contact, 66
Discharge Placement Meeting, 56

Early Permanence Placement (EPP), xiv, 6, 7, 16, 17, 36, 38, 39, 64, 88, 104, 113, 116, 185
emergency court hearing, 108, 116, 117
emergency hospital visits, 142
emotional triggers, 10

foetal alcohol spectrum disorders (FASDs), 37, 69
foster care, xiv, xviii, 3, 5, 6, 7, 11, 16, 31, 34, 48, 57, 71, 93, 105, 110, 143, 161, 187
Further Action on Adoption: Finding More Loving Homes, 5

Goodman Project, 4
guardian, xiv, 72, 105, 108, 109, 114, 115, 141, 166

health visitor assessment, 175
home assessment, 42, 43, 44, 45, 46, 47, 48, 49, 50, 51, 52, 53, 54, 55, 56, 57, 58, 59, 60, 61, 62, 63, 64, 65, 66, 67, 68, 69, 70, 71, 72

independent reviewing officer (IRO), xiv, 72, 114, 115, 168, 169, 172, 181, 186
Interim Care Order (ICO), xiv, 4, 71, 140, 161

LAC Review, 114, 141, 142, 147, 151, 167, 168, 169, 172, 181, 186, 195
Later Life letter, xiv, 52, 172, 186, 211
Letterbox contact, 34, 49
life story book, xv, 53, 103, 142, 158, 172, 175, 179, 180, 186, 203
Link Maker, xv, 36, 94, 203
Local Authority, xv, 3, 4, 5, 6, 7, 13, 18, 113, 135, 140, 141, 143, 160, 161, 185, 203
long-term impacts, 79
Looked After Child (LAC), xv, 136, 168, 172, 173, 190, 195, 203

Matching Panel, xv, 93, 96, 106, 116, 118, 120, 146, 157, 158, 159, 160, 161, 162, 163, 164, 165, 166, 167, 168, 169, 170, 171, 172, 173, 174, 175, 186
Mother and Baby Unit, xv, 71, 105, 161

PACE (playfulness, acceptance, curiosity, empathy) model, 35, 60, 66, 209

Pen Picture, xv, 59, 61
permanent long-term foster care, 31
Placement Order (PO), xv, 2, 5, 10, 44, 49, 74, 93, 119, 120, 140, 160, 162, 170, 171, 185, 201, 206
post-adoption support, 21
potential adopters, 22
Prospective Adopters Report (PAR), xv, 20, 28, 29, 40, 53, 64, 65, 93, 99

reassurance, 132, 184
relinquished children, xvi, 2, 7, 12, 15, 16, 17, 49, 96, 111, 114

secondary trauma, 67
social workers, 135, 142, 144, 146, 152
Special Care Baby Unit, 55, 110
Special Guardianship, 31
Special Guardianship assessment, 113
Special Guardianship Order, 85
Stage 1 adoption process, xvi, 20, 21, 27, 39, 40, 51
Stage 2 adoption process, xvi, 20, 22, 38, 39, 42, 43, 49, 62, 96, 156
stand-in contact supervisors, 141

terminated placement, 6, 8–9, 44, 45, 109–13
Theraplay, xvi, 51, 53